VASCULAR RESEARCH DEVELOPMENTS

PERIPHERAL ARTERY DISEASE

FROM RISK FACTORS
TO MANAGEMENT

VASCULAR RESEARCH DEVELOPMENTS

Additional books and e-books in this series can be found
on Nova's website under the Series tab.

VASCULAR RESEARCH DEVELOPMENTS

PERIPHERAL ARTERY DISEASE

FROM RISK FACTORS
TO MANAGEMENT

JEREMY D. PARKS
EDITOR

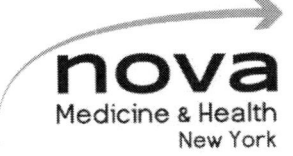

nova
Medicine & Health
New York

Library of Congress Cataloging-in-Publication Data

ISBN: 978-1-53619-968-0

Published by Nova Science Publishers, Inc. † New York

CONTENTS

PREFACE

Peripheral Artery Disease is a circulatory condition usually caused by the buildup of fatty deposits and calcium in the walls of the arteries. The condition is often painful and chronic but can be managed with lifestyle changes and medication. Chapter one describes the psychological factors associated with peripheral arterial disease. Chapter two describes how lifestyle changes play an important role in the management of diabetes and peripheral artery disease. Chapter three explains the role of the family physician in risk management of peripheral artery disease. Lastly, Chapter four focuses on questionnaires for primary care physicians, which can be used for peripheral arterial disease symptom screening and assessing functional impairment and quality of life of patients.

Chapter 1 - Peripheral arterial disease (PAD) is a global problem that is seen all over the world and is expected to increase in the following years. Although the disease has certain levels, it has an asymptomatic state as well as severe levels that can have more negative consequences for patients. There are also treatment modalities that may differ depending on the level of the disease. Not only patients but also family members are affected by the disease. There are many risk factors determined by studies for PAD. Interventions are also made for these risk factors. It is these risk factors that are tried to be changed for the first time in patients. Then, other treatments are started. Two important interventions for risk factors are smoking cessation and exercise. These two interventions are also included in this section. As a results of the PAD experiences, it has been stated that PAD was associated with the increase in depression and anxiety. In addition, the fact that this disease has an impact on the lives of patients brings along an impact on their quality of life and psychological health. In this sense, many studies have been carried out, and in this section, both these studies and the few interventions made in this sense are included within the scope of this section.

Chapter 2 - Diabetes, a serious threat for global health together with peripheral artery disease, became a burden for both patients and the health care systems for their social and economic consequences. Each of them is a predictor for the other, and even worsen the prognosis of the patient if they are present at the same time. As a coincidence both group of patients are unaware of their health status, which can progress towards a much serious problem ending with limb loss. The primary care physicians are important for the awareness of patients having diabetes and peripheral artery disease for their increased risk of comorbidity and complications that need follow up for appropriate diagnosis, treatment and referral when needed. In addition, it is important to keep in contact with these patients for their life style changes; nutritional behaviors, physical activities and exercise training, blood sugar monitoring and applying medications, risk reduction, problem solving abilities and need for seeking medical care. Often a successful diabetes education, will give the patients a real role in many dietary and lifestyle modifications thus improve self-care significantly, with the support of healthcare professionals, which gives them self-confidence that reduces the mortality and morbidity as well as health care costs and improves the health care quality of life.

Chapter 3 - Peripheral arterial disease (PAD) is a multifactorial process defined as a partial or complete occlusion of an artery in the upper or lower extremity due to atherosclerosis. It has similar risk factors to other cardiovascular diseases. The most important risk factors are diabetes mellitus, tobacco use, hypertension, and dyslipidemia. In addition, age, gender, ethnicity, inactivity and being overweight play a role. Since many people have asymptomatic PAD, known risk factors should be managed appropriately and in a timely manner. As a multifactorial disease, PAD requires multidimensional screening as well as easily applicable and accessible follow-up approaches. At this context, primary care physicians have an important position in screening undiagnosed asymptomatic PAD and in monitoring patients with explained increased cardiovascular risk due to PAD. Risk factors - Smoking increases risk of PAD up to a 10-fold. A systematic review suggests that half of all PADs are attributable to smoking. It was concluded that heavier smokers were more likely to develop PAD than light smokers, and that former smokers had a steadily increased risk compared to never smokers. Exposure to passive smoking has also been shown to promote changes leading to atherosclerosis. Diabetes has been shown to increase the risk of PAD 2-4 times. Poor diabetic control is associated with an increased risk of PAD. The risk of developing PAD is proportional to the severity and duration of diabetes. Dyslipidemia is correlated with accelerated PAD. Dyslipidemia management by diet, exercise, and/or medication is associated with a major reduction in cardiovascular diseases and stroke. Hypertension can increase risk of developing PAD. High blood pressure increases the risk of intermittent claudication, the most common symptom of PAD. Other risk factors can be listed as genetics leading to risk factors for PAD such as diabetes and hypertension but there have been no specific genes or gene mutations directly associated with them. The prevalence and outcome of peripheral artery disease shows differences with age and gender of the patients. Considering all these risk factors in the population, family physicians have also a crucial role to arise PAD awareness among patients and general population. Increased awareness could enable earlier, appropriate and effective management of PAD and adherence to secondary prevention strategies for the modification of PAD risk factors at primary health care settings. This section will review PAD risk management and the role of family physician in primary care.

Chapter 4 - The progressive atherosclerotic process is the principal cause of the development of peripheral arterial disease (PAD), and has risk factors in common with atherosclerosis, such as tobacco smoking, diabetes mellitus, dyslipidemia, hypertension and being over the age of 50. The prevalence of PAD, predictably increases with advancing age and the presence of diabetes, leading to a prodigious burden of disease, due to the morbidity and mortality of cardiovascular and cerebrovascular events. Primary healthcare is an important point of care for the screening of PAD patients, especially those who are asymptomatic. The early recognition of PAD is critically important and the role of the family physician particularly so in the prevention and early assessment of PAD, particularly with regard to risk factors such as diabetes, smoking. To identify at-risk patients in the "murky zone" the physician requires a number of complex approaches in daily work practice. Family physicians can identify these patients using instrumental measurements and if necessary can refer them for further investigation. In the long run, launching an applicable, easy screening program at primary care level makes PAD patients easier to diagnose, leading to earlier diagnosis and treatment, which will significantly improve both the patients' quality of life and life expectancy. In addition to reliable non-invasive diagnostic tests, such as the ankle-brachial pressure index (ABI) simple and easily applied self-assessment tools for the symptoms and performance of patients. This review focuses on questionnaires for primary care physicians, which can be used for PAD symptom screening, functional impairment and the quality of life of the patients, for example the Edinburgh Claudication Questionnaire (ECQ), Walking Impairment Questionnaire (WIQ), Vascular Quality of Life Questionnaire (VascuQoL), all of which are frequently used by other PAD related disciplines.

In: Peripheral Artery Disease
Editor: Jeremy D. Parks

ISBN: 978-1-53619-968-0
© 2021 Nova Science Publishers, Inc.

Chapter 1

PSYCHOLOGICAL AND BEHAVIORAL FACTORS, INTERVENTIONS AND PSYCHOLOGICAL HEALTH IN PERIPHERAL ARTERIAL DISEASE

Elçin Yorulmaz and Gülay Dirik
Psychology Department, Dokuz Eylul University, İzmir, Turkey

ABSTRACT

Peripheral arterial disease (PAD) is a global problem that is seen all over the world and is expected to increase in the following years. Although the disease has certain levels, it has an asymptomatic state as well as severe levels that can have more negative consequences for patients. There are also treatment modalities that may differ depending on the level of the disease. Not only patients but also family members are affected by the disease. There are many risk factors determined by studies for PAD. Interventions are also made for these risk factors. It is these risk factors that are tried to be changed for the first time in patients. Then, other treatments are started. Two important interventions for risk factors are smoking cessation and exercise. These two interventions are also included in this section. As a results of the PAD experiences, it has been stated that PAD was associated with the increase in depression and anxiety. In addition, the fact that this disease has an impact on the lives of patients brings along an impact on their quality of life and psychological health. In this sense, many studies have been carried out, and in this section, both these studies and the few interventions made in this sense are included within the scope of this section.

Keywords: peripheral arterial disease, risk factors, psychological distresses, quality of life

INTRODUCTION

There are 236.62 million patients with peripheral arterial disease (PAD) worldwide in 2015 (Song et al. 2019, e1020). In addition, 70.200 people died due to PAD in 2017 (James et al. 2018, 1789). In other words, PAD has been a global problem in the 21st century (Song et al. 2019, e1020) and prevalence has been increasing day by day (Sampson et al. 2014, 145). The definition of PAD is "an atherosclerotic disease of the non-cardiac vessels" (Creager et al. 2012). The severity of PAD can vary. The severity of PAD can be intermittent claudication with pain in lower extremities after exercise, as well as critical limb ischaemia in which rest pain, ulcers and gangrene can also be experienced (Aboyans et al. 2018, 795). It is stated that PAD has four categories. These categories are asymptomatic PAD, intermittent claudication, atypical exertional leg symptoms, and pain at rest. In addition, it was found that symptomatic PAD is less common than asymptomatic PAD (McDermott et al. 2013, e000257). While it was stated in previous studies that PAD was more common in men (Kröger et al. 2006, 279), it is now concluded that it is as common in women as men. Women are more often seen as asymptomatic or show atypical symptoms compared to men (Barochiner, Aparicio, & Waisman, 2014, 115). It is seen that the ankle-brachial index and 6 minute walk test are used as measurements in PAD patients. Ankle-brachial index was used to establish PAD diagnosis. 0,9 was considered as a threshold and it is inversely associated to atherosclerotic risk factors and the presence of cardiovascular and cerebrovascular diseases (Fowkes, 1988, 248). In addition, 6 minute walk test was found highly reliable measurement for PAD patients (Montgomery & Gardner, 1998, 706). In terms of treatment, PAD patients need to change their risk factors regardless of the level of their disease. Afterwards, drug treatments and exercises are recommended to the patients. If these methods do not work or if there is a worsening situation, patients are directed to revascularization, angioplasty or bypass surgery (Hiatt, 2001, 1612). When these methods are not effective, amputation can be suggested to patients, which is seen as the last alternative (Kolossvary et al. 2015, 83). In summary, PAD is a common condition and its prevalence is expected to increase. As the severity of the disease varies, there are also different representations. While it was concluded that its prevalence in men and women does not differ, it is seen that there are different tools in measurements and options for treatment.

Patients' Experiences with PAD

PAD patients may have different experiences as well as above characteristics of the disease. In a study, it was aimed to examine PAD patients' experiences of living with PAD. Within the scope of this study, 24 patients with different levels of PAD were interviewed. They stated that living with PAD is an effort to live and relax with a difficult physical, social and emotional burden. It has been stated that the themes that arise about experiencing burden are being restricted by the burden, trying to relax from the burden, accepting the feeling of burden and adapting to this feeling. It has been stated that it is important to use different coping strategies to provide relief. It was concluded that pain and sleep are the main characteristics associated with living with PAD. It has been stated that pain-related education and pain management are important for the relief of pain (Wann-Hansson et al. 2005, 851). In another study, it was also aimed to examine the experiences of patients living with PAD. In this context, a systematic review was made and 14 studies with 360 participants were included in the study. Although patients have different symptoms, they experience pain and walking limitation. It has been reported that ignoring the symptoms of the patients delayed their diagnosis. In addition, inadequate engagement regarding the disease and treatment options may be related to the poor attitudes for walking treatments and unrealistic expectations about surgery. It is stated that depending on the progression of the symptoms, patients may have problems in walking, feel weak and lose their independence, which may be the source of the burden for them. It is stated that not being able to understand the disease sufficiently is at the center of PAD, and even if the patients get used to living with this disease for a long time, they have concerns about their future (Abaraogu et al. 2018, e0207456). In addition to examining the experiences of the patients during the illness, the experiences of the patients during the treatments were also examined by the studies. For example, one study examined long-term experiences with the healing process after revascularization. In this study, interviews were conducted with 14 patients 6 months and 2.5 years after revascularization. It has been stated that while living with PAD for the long term, individuals become aware of their chronic illness over time. First of all, individuals stated that they perceived this as an acute condition, then they went to the recovery phase after revascularization, and finally they went to the chronic phase of PAD. In the stage where they perceive PAD as chronic, they stated that they did not recover but got better, took control over their lives again, and reevaluated the meaning of life (Wann-Hansson et al. 2008, 552). In another study where participants' experiences with amputation were examined, 33 interviews were conducted. These interviews were conducted with vascular patients living in lower limb amputation at tibia, knee, or femoral level. The amputation process has been examined in 3 stages. These stages are the decision stage, surgical intervention stage and rehabilitation stage. Content analysis was conducted on these stages and 3 themes emerged. The themes "from irreversible problem to amputation decision" during the decision phase, "a feeling of being in a vacuum" during the surgical intervention, and "adaptation to new life" during the rehabilitation phase emerged. The patients stated that they felt abandoned during the surgical procedure. It was concluded that most of the participants were satisfied with these decisions, while some participants regretted not having an amputation before. It has been stated that it is important to develop a partnership with the surgeon so that the patients feel part of the care for their well-being. In addition, it was stated that patients need to be informed about the whole process and thus they are better prepared for the whole process. It is stated that it may be beneficial to present amputation as a valuable treatment option earlier in order to increase the quality of life of patients and reduce unnecessary suffering (Torbjörnsson et al. 2017, 57).

Considering the experiences of PAD patients, treatments and restricted life, it seems inevitable that family members also affected by this situation. In a study, interviews were conducted with 10 spouses whose spouses experienced intermittent claudication. These themes are "frustrating to not meet intentions, undergoing changes in social life, being a person on the side of things, intertwining of circumstances." It is stated that the dominant theme is "living a demanding life." Intermittent claucidation has important effects on the daily lives of the spouses as well as the patient's life, and it is difficult to live with intermittent claudication patients (Egberg et al. 2013, 610). In another study, 7 PAD patients and their caregivers were included. Their experiences in this process was handled. While PAD patients stated that pain was central in their experience with PAD, they stated that their movements were restricted and they lost their independence. While patients stated that they needed an understanding of their illnesses, caregivers also stated that they needed to feel accepted for their roles (Johnstone 2004, 36).

In summary, the experiences of patients during PAD and after various procedures and the experiences of family members and caregivers have been examined in different studies. To put it briefly, PAD is a condition that affects not only patients but also the lives of family members as well as caregivers.

Risk Factors for PAD

It is stated that risk factors for PAD are age, level of fibrinogen (Meijer et al. 2000, 2934) smoking, diabetes, hypertension, hypercholesterolaemia (Meijer et al. 2000, 2934, Song et al., 2019, e1020), and obesity (Huang et al. 2016, 218). In addition, PAD was found to be associated with coronary hearth disease (Murabito et al. 2002, 961). According to gender, it was claimed that women and men were not different in terms of risk factors for PAD (Meijer et al. 2000, 2934). In line with the risk factors found, 4,470 men aged 65 to 83 participated in a study. It was determined that 744 of the participants were PAD. The main risk factor is increased age, past or present smoking, physical inactivity, a history of angina, and diabetes mellitus. While the highest risk is stated to be using 25 or more cigarettes a day, it has been stated that smoking was also an important risk factor in the past, even if not using it now (Fowler et al. 2007, 219). In another study comparing men with PAD with men without PAD, men without PAD less likely to have hypertension, diabetes mellitus, a history of smoking, a better lipid profile and lower levels of inflammatory biomarkers as compared to men with PAD (Grenon et al. 2014, 396). In another comparative study, the findings were similar. Individuals with a diagnosis of PAD are reported to smoke frequently, have the lowest smoking cessation rates, are less physically active, frequently have a previous diagnosis of diabetes, and report higher blood pressure levels compared to individuals without PAD. It is stated that individuals with suspected PAD have higher smoking cessation rates but higher rates of obesity compared to patients without PAD (Reiner et al. 2021, 227). In summary, age, fibrinogen level, smoking, diabetes, hypertension, hypercholesterolaemia, coronary heart disease, obesity and sedentary life seem to be risk factors for PAD. Now, these risk factors will be studied in detail.

In a study on diabetes, participants were examined for diabetes and PAD for 12 years. While men with diabetes have been reported to have a higher risk of PAD compared to men without diabetes, the duration of diabetes also increases the risk of developing PAD (Al-Delaimy et al. 2004, 236). Similarly, in another study, it is stated that diabetes increases the risk of PAD (Marso & Hiatt, 2006, 921). PAD is common in diabetic patients and this prevalence increases with age (Faglia, 2011, 152). As diabetes increases risk, the duration of diabetes and age appear to be important for developing PAD. While the American Diabetes Association has also published a commentaries on PAD in diabetes patients (American Diabetes Association, 2003, 3333), review studies have been conducted on peripheral arterial disease in diabetes patients (Jude, Eleftheriadou, & Tentolouris, 2010, 4). In addition to examining diabetes, patients with coronary heart disease have been studied. In this study performed with 8243 coronary heart disease patients, intermittent claucidation is common in coronary heart patients, but PAD also increases the risk of coronary heart disease (Reiner et al. 2021, 227). Similarly, in another study, it was concluded that individuals with PAD are more likely to have coronary heart disease and cerebrovascular disease compared to individuals without PAD (Criqui et al. 1997, 221). In conclusion, diabetes and coronary heart disease appear to be associated with PAD.

In a study, the relationship between body mass index and PAD was examined. 3,250,350 individuals participated in the study and 27.8% of the participants were stated to be obese. It was found a J shaped relationship between body mass index and prevalence of PAD. It means that underweight was related to higher prevalence of PAD. Overweight individuals showed the lowest prevalence of PAD. In addition, obesity was related to PAD especially for women, this relation was weaker for men (Heffron et al. 2020, 31). Similar to this study, the relationship between body mass index and PAD was investigated in a study. It was concluded that there was a U shaped relationship between them. While both obesity and being underweight are reported to be associated with PAD, overweight was not related to PAD (Desormais et al. 2019, 50). In parallel with the finding that obesity is a risk factor, it has been concluded that obesity and underweight increase the risk of PAD while examining the relationship between body mass index and PAD in these studies.

As the body mass index is examined, the relationship between nutrition, which can be considered as a related factor, with PAD has been examined by studies. While no relationship was found between fruit and vegetable consumption and PAD in one study (Hung et al. 2003, 659), other studies found that the Mediterranean diet (Ruiz-Canela et al. 2014, 415) and nut consumption (Heffron et al. 2015, 15) reduces the possibility of developing PAD. In another study, meat consumption increased the risk of developing PAD, low alcohol intake and coffee consumption increased the risk of developing PAD (Ogilvie et al. 2017, 651). In a study involving 1592 men and women, the relationship between nutrition and PAD was examined. It has been stated that fiber-containing foods are associated with a higher ankle brachial index for men, while consuming high-level meat and meat-related products is associated with a low ankle brachial index for both men and women. Additionally, it was concluded that cereal fiber and alcohol were positively associated with the ankle brachial index in men (Donnan et al. 1993, 917). Another study included 46,032 men aged between 40 and 75 years. Participants were followed for 12 years and it was aimed to examine the relationship between dietary fiber and PAD. While the participants were not PAD at the beginning, at the end of 12 years 308 participants had PAD. Fruit, vegetable and total fiber intakes were not related to incidence of PAD. However, there was found an inverse relationship between cereal fiber and the risk of PAD. It has been concluded that increased consumption of cereal fiber may prevent the formation of PAD (Merchant et al. 2003, 3658). In another study, the relationship between Mediterranean diet and asymptomatic PAD in premenopausal women was examined. It was found that low adherence to Mediterranean Diet is related to low ankle branchial index, indicator of asymptomatic atherosclerosis (Mattioli et al. 2017, 985). In summary, it was stated that the Mediterranean type of diet, nut and cereal fiber consumption may reduce the risk, while high meat consumption may increase the risk.

The role of alcohol consumption and smoking for PAD were also examined in the studies. It is observed that the risk of PAD is frequently examined with the amount of alcohol associated with alcohol consumption. For example, in one study, participants were grouped according to their alcohol consumption amount as never, occasional, mild, moderate and heavy. It was concluded that moderate alcohol use was associated with a lower prevalence compared to no alcohol use. Heavy alcohol use has been reported to be associated with the increase in the prevalence of PAD (Athyros et al. 2007, 689). In a study with male physicians, participants were followed for 11 years and it was concluded that moderate alcohol consumption reduced the risk of PAD (Camargo et al. 1997, 577). In another study, 1.937.360 individuals were followed for about 6 years. During this time, 114,859 of them were diagnosed with cardiovascular disease. It was concluded that no alcohol consumption increases the risk of PAD compared to moderate use, but the risk of PAD increases for heavy users (Bell et al. 2017, 1). In a study with 3795 participants, the relationship between alcohol consumption and PAD was examined. It was found that there is an inverse relationship between moderate alcohol consumption and PAD for women. This association was not confirmed for men (Vliegenthart et al. 2002, 332). In another study, age and gender matched 56,544 adult with alcohol intoxication and 226,176 person without alcohol intoxication were compared. It was concluded that alcohol intoxication increased the incidence of PAD (Huang et al. 2017, 25). Based on these studies, it can be concluded that no alcohol consumption and heavy use of alcohol increase the risk, while moderate use decreases the risk.

In studies conducted in terms of smoking, it is observed that the relationship between smoking levels and PAD was examined, comparing smokers with non-smokers PAD patients, and examining the concept of passive smoking in this context. In a study comparing moderate and heavy smokers with those who never smoked, it was concluded that smoking is a strong risk factor for PAD (Price et al. 1999, 344). In another study, patients with PAD who smoke and individuals who smoke but do not have PAD were compared. It was concluded that smoking, with higher cigarette exposure and the highest nicotine yield, increased the risk of smokers to develop PAD. In addition, the presence of hypertension in smokers also increases the risk of developing PAD (Powell et al. 1997, 41). In addition to these comparison studies, the relationship between passive smoking and PAD, as stated, was also examined. In this context, the concept of second hand smoke was handled. This is defined as smoking exposure at home or at work, even though people do not smoke. It was concluded that second hand smoke and PAD are related, and the prevalence of PAD increases with the increase in exposure to second hand smoke. Based on these findings, it appears that not only smoking but also passive smoking is a risk factor for PAD (He et al. 2008, 1535). When studies conducted in terms of smoking are examined, it is concluded that increased use or exposure increases the risk of PAD.

In addition to considering smoking and alcohol as a risk factor, it has been tried to determine the related factors in reducing their use, that is, in the development of health behaviors. For example, one study examined alcohol misuse and smoking in individuals experiencing amputation due to PAD. Before and 12 months after amputation, individuals were evaluated within the scope of alcohol misuse and smoking. 75 veterans participated in this study. While 16% of the participants reported alcohol misuse before the surgery, 13% reported alcohol misuse 12 months after the surgery. When evaluated in terms of smoking, 37% of the participants smoked before the surgery, this number decreased to 29% 12 months after the surgery. When the participants whose alcohol use decreased and who quit smoking are examined, it is seen that these participants report high levels of social support. It has been stated that the presence of social support can encourage individuals to change their health behavior (Turner et al. 2014, 494). In summary, smoking and alcohol use emerges as a risk factor, and social support seems to have a protective role in terms of alcohol misuse and smoking.

Finally, it appears that the role of the level of mobility is also examined in PAD patients. In a study, the relationship between sedentary time and PAD was examined and it was stated that sedentary time and PAD are related, but this relationship occurs when sedentary time is high. In other words, when the threshold is exceeded for sedentary time, the probability of PAD increases (Unkart et al. 2020, 208). In another study, the relationship between physical activity and PAD was examined. It was concluded that more exercise at 35-45 years of age in males was associated with less likelihood of PAD. For men and women between the ages of 55-74, higher levels of exercise at age 35-45 years were found to be related to lower blood viscosity and plasma fibrinogen levels. The ankle brachial pressure index of men between the ages of 55-74 who smoke in any period of their lives is associated with leisure activities between the ages of 35-45. Based on this finding, it has been suggested that physical activity in the early middle age may have a protective role in terms of PAD, especially for male smokers (Housley et al. 1993, 475). In summary, it appears that physical activity has a protective role for PAD and that increasing levels of sedentary life may increase the risk of PAD.

In conclusion, age, diabetes, coronary heart disease, body mass index, nutrition, smoking, alcohol use and inactivity are risk factors for PAD. Studies have examined these risk factors and the variables associated with these factors.

Interventions for PAD

There are many intervention studies aimed at changing these risk factors (e.g., Chi & Jaff, 2008, 475, Parvar et al. 2018, 1595, Verma et al. 2011, 34). In a study, a protocol was created for changing lifestyle and risk factors. Half of the participants will participate in the risk factor modification intervention program at the community-based center within the intervention group, while the other half will receive standard health care advice as a control group. The intervention is a 12-week, nurse-led, community-based, lifestyle and risk factor modification program. It consists of two phases and is based on the use of pharmacotherapy, which supports nutrition, exercise and lifestyle changes. It was stated that this study will show the effectiveness of the lifestyle and risk factor modification intervention program (Elfghi et al. 2021, 1-2). With a pilot study in which participants 'self-management was supported, an intervention was conducted to improve participants' health behaviors. Participants had a 50-minute evaluation session with the health psychologist, this session was conducted individually. The intervention is called low intensity, the reason why it is called low intensity depends on the number of face-to-face sessions with the healthcare professional.

Within the scope of this study, lower face-to-face interviews were made, and follow-up interviews were carried out by phone and e-mail. Health psychologists have focused on why health is important to them, what they want to change, and what they want to be different over the 6-month period. Motivational interview approach was used. Participants received an activity tracker to record their daily number of steps, and psychological input was provided on weekly goal setting, overcoming obstacles and preventing relapse. Participants were evaluated at the beginning, 3 months later, and 6 months later. It was reported that depression scores improved significantly when the initial measures were compared with those 6 months later. It was reported that 8 of the 23 participants who were followed for 6 months stopped smoking, and an additional 9 participants reduced their use. In addition, it was stated that there was an increase in daily step count in the follow-up 6 months later compared to the baseline. Participants emphasized that they understand and embrace the information given about the importance of changing health behaviors (McCallum et al. 2020, 1). In summary, protocols have been developed for changing risk factors and improving health behaviors, as well as intervention studies.

In conclusion, interventions are made both to change these risk factors and to improve health behaviors. While this section deals with general interventions to change risk factors, the next section included interventions for specific risk factors. In this context, smoking cessation and exercise (Mukherjee & Yadav, 2001, 723), which are stated to be two important treatments for PAD, were handled.

Smoking Cessation Intervention for PAD

Smoking emerges as a risk factor for PAD as stated in the previous section. Many studies have been conducted on the relationship between smoking and PAD. In a meta-analysis study, it was concluded that there is a significant relationship between smoking and PAD. While the risk was stated to be less in former users, even this low risk was stated to be higher than those who never smoked (Lu, Mackay & Pell, 2014, 414). Similarly, in another study, it was stated that the risk of PAD for smokers was increased, even the risk was higher for former users. It has been reported that there is a dose-response relationship between smoking and PAD, and the risk increases significantly in heavy smokers (Willigendael et al. 2004, 1158). Other studies have also found that there is a dose-response relationship (Conen et al. 2011, 719, He et al. 2006, 333). Studies examining smoking in patients with PAD emphasize the need for smoking cessation interventions (Lu, Mackay & Pell, 2014, 414, Willigendael et al. 2004, 1158). Smoking cessation interventions significantly reduce the risk of PAD (Conen et al. 2011, 719). In addition to reducing the risk of PAD, PAD patients quitting smoking after PAD has important gains. It has been concluded that PAD patients who quit smoking report lower mortality compared to PAD patients who continue to smoke, and that their amputation-free survival is also increased (Armstrong et al. 2014, 1565). In summary, although smoking is a risk factor for PAD, cessation of smoking decreases the risk of PAD and can be associated with a more positive process for PAD patients.

Physician advice, nicotine replacement therapy, and bupropion are stated to be evidence-based interventions that increase the likelihood of smoking cessation (Hobbs & Bradbury, 2003, 341). In an intervention study on PAD patients who are smokers, the participants were randomly assigned to the intensive tailored PAD specific counseling intervention or minimal intervention group. Intensive intervention includes both physician advice and smoking cessation counseling. Counseling intervention consists of behavioral and pharmacological elements that are evidence-based for the general population of smoking. Counseling includes training on the relationship between smoking and the onset and progression of PAD, motivational interview to increase motivation for smoking cessation, cognitive behavioral counseling to develop a cessation plan, and information on pharmacological assistance used for smoking cessation. Counselors use problem-solving skills training and cognitive behavioral elements to help identify individual behavioral and cognitive strategies to cope with cigarette cravings, and to choose a date for cessation preparation and cessation goal. In addition, the participants were encouraged to choose an individual from their social environment who would support their quitting efforts. If the participant has permission, the counselors also provided information on how to support this selected person. While 6 consultancy sessions are planned to be held over a 5-month period, the first meeting will be held face-to-face, and subsequent interviews are planned to be held face to face or over the phone, depending on the availability of the participants. Participants in the minimal intervention group only received verbal advice about quitting smoking. Measurements were taken from the participants before and 3 months and 6 months after the intervention. It was concluded that the participants in the intensive intervention group had higher non-smoking rates in their follow-up evaluations 6 months later (Hennrikus et al. 2010, 2105-2112). In another study, participants were randomly assigned to the intervention and control groups. Participants in the intervention group received brief smoking cessation counseling, medications, and quit line referrals. Measurements were taken from the participants after clinic visits and 3 months later. While 156 participants completed the first measurements, 75 participants completed the measurements 3 months later. Participants in both the intervention group and the control group stated that they had unsuccessful smoking cessation attempts. Compared to the control group receiving standard care, the participants in the intervention group stated that they received more advice from their surgeons about quitting and had some or a lot interest in quitting. In addition, participants in the intervention group tend to acknowledge addictive behaviors and the negative health consequences of smoking. In the measurements taken 3 months after the intervention, it was concluded that the participants in the intervention group had a greater reduction in nicotine addiction (Newhall et al. 2017, 113).

In summary, smoking is an important risk factor for PAD. It is very important to stop smoking in order to prevent the occurrence of PAD and to make PAD patients experience less negativity. Therefore, there are studies conducted in this sense and the results of these studies point to positive results for PAD patients.

Exercise Intervention for PAD

Risk factors were mentioned in the previous section. Inactivity and obesity appear to be a risk factor, and interventions to change risk factors in general were briefly mentioned. However, it is striking that studies on exercise intervention have an important place in the literature. Exercise interventions will be discussed in detail in this section.

It is seen that an intervention in the sense of exercise is supervised exercise training. In a study conducted, the effects of supervised exercise training applied for 6 months and 12 months on strength and endurance parameters in PAD patients were evaluated. 94 participants were included in the study, 42 of them completed the 6-month training program, and 52 of them completed the 12-month protocol. Significant increases were observed in the parameters evaluated in pushing, pulling, and tiptoe standing in both groups. However, those in the 12-month group benefited more. In both groups, absolute claudication distance increased similarly. However, walking speed increased for 12 month group more than 6 month group (Pilz et al. 2014, 383). In one study, a pilot exercise intervention was performed to improve lower extremity functioning of PAD patients who did not show intermittent claudication. Within the scope of the study, 32 female and male participants were randomly assigned to exercise training or usual care groups. Participants in the intervention group showed greater improvements in their Walking Impairment Questionnaire walking speed scores, 6-minute walk distance, maximal treadmill walking distance, the Walking Impairment Questionnaire's distance score, and the Walking Impairment Questionnaire's speed score compared to the control group. Based on this finding, it was concluded that the supervised treadmill walking program increased the functionality of PAD patients without intermittent claudication symptoms (McDermott et al. 2004, 187). In another study, supervised walking therapy was found to be effective for increasing walking distance and pain-free walking distance in patients with intermittent claudication (Fakhry et al. 2012, 1132). Although the positive results of supervised walking therapy have been shown in this study, participation in supervised exercise programs poses a serious problem

(Harwood et al. 2016, 280). In summary, while supervised exercise programs show positive results in terms of increasing the mobility of the participants, it was emphasized that participation constitutes an important problem.

In addition to supervised exercise programs, the relationship between PAD diagnosis and exercise-based cardiac rehabilitation was examined in a study. While 23,215 patients participated in the study, 1366 of these patients were reported to be PAD. Participants were directed to a 12-week exercise-based cardiac rehabilitation program. It was concluded that PAD patients had a lower inclination to start cardiac rehabilitation and to complete it if they did. It was stated that PAD patients who completed Cardiac rehabilitation had lower exercise capacity at the beginning and after the rehabilitation was completed. While 3510 deaths were experienced in follow-up measurements, 10 year survival was found to be lower for patients with PAD. In addition, completion of cardiac rehabilitation was related to lower mortality. It was stated that these findings also support the use of cardiac rehabilitation in PAD patients (Devrome et al. 2019, 108). In parallel with what happened in the supervised exercise program, it was stated that participation in cardiac rehabilitation was a problem, but exercise-based cardiac rehabilitation also had positive effects for the participants.

It is also seen that cognitive behavioral approaches are used in terms of exercise. In a study, 6 month group mediated cognitive behavioral intervention was performed for PAD patients. Participants were randomized to the group mediated cognitive behavioral intervention or control group. The first phase of the research lasts from the 1st to the 6th month. The intervention was in the form of weekly internet meetings that used group support and self-regulation skills to increase participants' participation in home-based exercise. The control group, on the other hand, received weekly online lessons on subjects unrelated to exercise. At the end of the first phase, the measurement was taken. In the second phase, which lasted from the 7th to the 12th month, the groups were contacted over the phone. Compared to the control group, the 6 minute walk distance and walking impairment questionnaire speed score of the intervention group increased at 12 months follow up compared to the first measurement. However, in the follow-up measurement at the end of 12 months, the two groups do not differ in terms of the walking impairment questionnaire distance score. Based on these findings, it was concluded that the participants continued to benefit from the 12-month follow-up measurements 6 months after the intervention ended (McDermott et al. 2014, e000711). The same study was also evaluated in terms of mobility loss. Compared to the control group, fewer participants in the intervention group experienced mobility loss at the 6-month follow-up measurement and the 12-month follow-up measurement (McDermott et al. 2015, e001659). In another study, the effects of home based group mediated cognitive behavioral walking intervention on participants' self efficacy for walking, desire for physical competence, satisfaction of physical functioning, social functioning and acceptance of PAD related pain and discomfort were examined. For this reason, 194 PAD patients who participated in the study were randomized to home based group mediated cognitive behavioral walking intervention or attention control condition. Participants in the intervention group had a meeting with other PAD patients once a week, these group discussions were led by a facilitator. The sessions last about 90 minutes, 45 of these 90 minutes are discussed under the direction of the facilitator, and 45 minutes are walking exercise. Reviewing PAD in the sessions, providing information on the benefits of walking exercise for PAD patients, goal setting, self-monitoring, and pain management during exercise. 178 of the participants completed their first measurements and 6-month follow-up measurements. In the follow-up evaluation 6 months after the treatment, it was concluded that the intervention group had greater improvements in self-efficacy, satisfaction with functionality, pain acceptance, and social functionality compared to the control group (Rejeski et al. 2014, 1).

Internet-based and telephone-based interventions are also being developed to enable PAD patients to walk regularly (Kumar et al. 2018, 23). Additionally, protocols for brief behavioral interventions are created to increase the physical activity of the participants. For example, while 200 PAD patients are expected to participate in a study, participants will be randomly assigned to the intervention or control group. Both groups will receive a written paper on PAD management that includes usual medical care, 4 individualized interactions with the healthcare professional over a 3-month period, and walking advice. The control group will make four 15-minute phone calls including general discussion of PAD symptoms, health and well-being. The intervention group will receive behavioral counseling in the form of 2 times 1 hour face-to-face sessions and 2 times 15 minutes phone calls. This study was prepared in the form of a protocol, and it was stated that this study would evaluate the efficacy of brief behavioral counseling intervention in PAD patients with significant load (Burton et al. 2016, 1-2). In summary, it is seen that cognitive-behavioral elements are also used in exercise interventions for PAD patients, and innovations for these programs are also being tried to be created.

It is seen that many exercise interventions have been done so far. Due to the current COVID-19 pandemic, the impact of these interventions on COVID-19 has also been examined. For example, in one study, participants participated in the structured in-home walking program before the COVID-19 pandemic. After this program, there was a lockdown and during this process, it was examined whether the participants continued their mobility regarding this program while their movements were limited. Participants were evaluated at hospital visits approximately once a month. Information about the program is provided and the program consists of 8-minute walking sessions 2 times a day, 6 days a week. According to the evaluations, changes in the duration or intensity of these sessions are made. During the lockdown period, the rehabilitation team provided telephone support. Measurements were taken from the participants at their last hospital visits before the lockdown and on their return to the hospital after the lockdown. Participants' 6 minute walking distance remained constant, while their pain-free walking distance improved. However, while participants with less than 3 months of the intervention had an improvement in 6 minutes and pain free walking distances, it was concluded that the assessments of participants more than 3 months were stable. While there was a decrease in the body weights of the participants, there was no change in their blood pressure and ankle-brachial indexes.

However, these values are better for participants less than 3 months into the intervention (Lamberti et al. 2021, 1).

In summary, it is seen that many exercise interventions are performed to increase positive results in PAD patients. While there are many different applications, it is striking that protocols for development have also been prepared in recent years. In addition, whether COVID-19, which is a pandemic today, has an effect on these interventions has also been handled in the studies.

Psychological Health:
Psychological Distresses and Quality of Life in PAD

PAD is associated with psychological distresses such as depression and anxiety (Aragao et al. 2019, 1, Columbo et al. 2016, 235, Smolderen et al. 2009, 297), it has been concluded that the prevalence of depressive disorders increases as the severity of the disease increases (Wong et al. 2007, 471). In addition to PAD being associated with depression and anxiety, it is seen that there are studies comparing individuals with and without PAD in the context of depression. For example, in a study comparing women with PAD and women without PAD, women without PAD were less likely to be depressed as compared to women with PAD (Grenon et al. 2014, 396). It is stated that PAD patients are more likely to experience depression, even if their disease is asymptomatic (Toth-Vajna et al. 2020, 1). Similarly, another study compared individuals aged 55 and over with and without PAD. It has been concluded that individuals with PAD experience depressive mood two times more frequently than individuals without PAD (Arseven et al. 2001, 229). As a result, in addition to the fact that PAD is associated with depression and anxiety, it is seen that individuals with PAD are more likely to experience depression compared to individuals without PAD.

In addition to the comparison studies, the prevalence of psychological distresses in PAD patients was also examined. In a study, it was concluded that 29% of the participants had anxiety, 30% had depression and 28% had anhedonia (Smolderen et al. 2009, 297). In another study conducted with PAD patients, measurements of depression, anxiety, and stress were taken from 1,215 participants who participated in the study. It is stated that 51.1% of the participants reported symptoms higher than at least one of these measurements, 9.6% from two and 6.1% from three measurements. When evaluated based on symptoms, 16% of the participants reported high levels of depression, 10% of anxiety, and 46.8% of perceived stress (Thomas et al. 2018, A2040). Apart from cross-sectional studies, longitudinal studies were also conducted to determine the prevalence of psychological symptoms of PAD patients. In a longitudinal study, it was concluded that the prevalence of depression or depressive symptoms varied between 3-36% (Brostow et al. 2017, 181). In another study, PAD patients were followed up for 18 months for depressive symptoms. In the initial measurements, it was stated that 16% of the patients reported depressive symptoms, while it was stated that the patients who were depressed had more pain and their walking distance was less. At the end of 18 months, it was concluded that the depressive symptoms of the patients who were mainly depressed did not change, 58% of the participants did not report depressive symptoms, 27% reported subclinical and 15% clinically manifest depressive symptoms (Smolderen et al. 2008, 27). In another study, the effect of depressive symptoms of PAD patients on their functionality over time was examined. 417 PAD patients were followed up once a year for 2 years. Enduring and new incidence of depressive symptoms were found to be related to greater decline in functional performance annually (Ruo et al. 2007, 415). In addition to examining depression longitudinally, another study also examines anxiety and stress. It was stated that the participants reported high levels of stress in both the first measurement and the measurement after 12 months, followed by depression and anxiety (Thomas et al. 2020, 109963). In summary, the prevalence of psychological distresses in PAD patients was examined, as well as the change and effects of these prevalence over time.

The fact that PAD increases the possibility of experiencing depression and is seen to be common raises the question of who are more likely to experience depression. It has been stated that depressed PAD patients are more likely to be female and African American and have more severe PAD symptoms and lower physical functioning (Brostow et al. 2017, 181). In another study, it was stated that being woman, married or in a permanent relationship, having a low monthly income, being alcoholic and having high blood pressure are associated with depression (Aragao et al. 2019, 1). In the context of personality traits, it is stated that type D personality increases the risk of depressive symptoms (Aquarius et al. 2007, 662). In another study, the relationship between cognitive coping and depressive symptoms in PAD patients was examined. Participants using rumination and catastrophizing as cognitive coping with disabilities were noted to report more depressive symptoms, while coping by seeking and re-engaging in alternative, meaningful goals were associated with less depressive symptoms (Garnefski et al. 2009, 132). In a study examining the relationship between coping and depression, in addition to cognitive coping, it was concluded that PAD patients using active coping strategies reported less depressive symptoms (Diaconescu & Diaconescu, 2017, 296). In addition to these studies, those who can go further (Arseven et al. 2001, 229), those who have more social support (Diaconescu & Diaconescu, 2017, 296), and those who experience lower impairment in lower extremity functioning (McDermott et al. 2003, 461), it is stated that they are less likely to experience depressive symptoms.

As the factors related to depression are examined, it is observed that there are studies that determine the factors related to anxiety, stress and mental health concern in general. While it was stated that anxiety and monthly income, smoking and high blood pressure were related (Aragao et al. 2019, 1), it was stated that those with atypical leg symptoms were twice as likely to experience anxiety (Smolderen et al. 2009, 297). Depression and anxiety are also examined, and they are considered together in some studies. For example, in a study, it was stated that participants with pain at rest reported anxiety, depression, and anhedonia (Smolderen et al. 2009, 297). In another study, participants who reported high levels of depression, anxiety, or perceived stress were younger, female, had less social support, and had a history of coronary artery disease, heart failure, or sleep apnea (Thomas et al. 2018, A2040). Similarly, it has been concluded that patients with mental health concerns are often female, young, individuals with more physical distress, less social support, and perceive worse health conditions (Thomas et al. 2020, 109963). In summary, as the factors related to depression were determined in the studies, the factors related to anxiety were also tried to be determined, and it was observed that there were studies that address psychological distress together.

Psychological distresses were examined as a risk factor for PAD, as well as the factors associated with the psychological distress experience of PAD patients. For example, a study conducted with an electronic health record of 1,937,360 patients revealed that depression is a risk factor for the development of PAD (Daskalopoulou et al. 2016, e0153838). In one study, individuals without PAD were followed for approximately 9.7 years. It is stated that 854 of 12.965 middle-aged participants have developed PAD. While it is stated that anger proneness and depressive symptoms are related in this development, perceived social support has no effect. In other words, individuals' high anger proneness and depressive symptoms emerges as a risk factor for developing PAD (Wattanakit et al. 2005, 199). Apart from PAD, it is stated that depression has a negative effect on walking ability and physical functioning (Brostow et al. 2017, 181). Similarly, in another study, it was concluded that there is a negative relationship between depressive symptoms and 6 minute walking distance. In other words, as depressive symptoms increased, 6 minute walking distance decreased (McDermott et al. 2003, 461). In parallel with these findings, it was concluded that depression is related to poor functional and surgical outcomes in individuals with PAD (Ramirez, Drudi, & Grenon, 2018, 478). In a study, it was aimed to determine the psychological factors associated with the functional recovery of PAD patients after lower extremity bypass. It was concluded that the recovery of the participants after the intervention was related to the depression level and social support (Wongkongkam et al. 2019, 3). In another study, it is seen that depression and anxiety are taken together. In a study with patients with intermittent claudication, participants presented depressive signs showed shorter pain-free walking distance and total walking distance than participants without signs of depression. This finding was similar in participants with and without anxiety. Participants who report depressive signs report more barriers to physical activity than those who do not. This finding is not valid for anxiety. In other words, depression can both create a negativity in terms of walking distance and create an obstacle to participation in physical activity (Ragazzo et al. 2020, e1802). In a study examining anxiety, it was concluded that anxiety increases the possibility of cardiovascular disease, while more studies are required to make such an inference for PAD (Batelaan et al. 2016, 228). In summary, while depression appears to be a risk factor for developing PAD, depression may also have negative effects on walking distances and physical functionality of patients. However, it is highlighted that more studies are needed for anxiety.

Psychological distresses levels of PAD patients can also be evaluated after the procedures. In a study, participants were evaluated within the scope of depression, anxiety, and need for information before and after hospital discharge after peripheral arterial bypass surgery. It was concluded that patients reported low-level anxiety and depression, and that they needed information to understand, prevent, and manage complications (Galloway et al. 1995, 35). In addition, the levels of depression and anxiety were examined by comparing the participants with coronary heart disease and PAD and those with coronary heart disease but without PAD. It is stated that those with coronary heart disease and PAD report higher anxiety and depression compared to those with coronary heart disease but not PAD (Reiner et al. 2021, 227).

Intervention studies have also been established for the psychological distresses of PAD patients. For example, for improving depression, cognitive behavioral self-help program was generated. In this study, it was stated that such an intervention had not been performed in PAD patients before (Garnefski et al. 2013, 186). Although there are no psychological intervention studies for psychological symptoms in PAD patients (Garnefski et al. 2013, 187), it has been seen that short psychological interventions are performed to increase the daily walking amount of PAD patients. In this sense, 58 PAD patients who participated in a study were randomly assigned to standard care and short psychological intervention groups. Participants in the standard care group received standard care and researcher interaction, while the intervention group received standard care and brief psychological intervention to establish a personalized walking plan and change beliefs about the disease and walking. The psychological intervention was carried out in the homes of the participants in two 1-hour sessions. The basic measurement is the daily step number of the participants, measured with a pedometer after 4 months. In the follow-up measurements 4 months after the intervention, it was concluded that the participants in the intervention group walked more daily than the control group (Cunnigham et al. 2012, 854). After this study, whether this change continued for 2 years was examined in another study. It was concluded that the participants in the intervention group still walked more than the control group in the measurements at the end of the 1st year and the 2nd year. Based on these studies, it was concluded that the change in the beliefs of PAD patients about illness and walking and having an individualized walking plan increased walking behavior and this increase was maintained for 2 years (Cunnigham et al. 2013, 756).

As a result, it is seen that PAD is associated with psychological distresses, may appear as a risk factor for developing PAD, and may be associated with experiencing more negativity related to the disease. In this context, it is seen that the interventions are important.

PAD and Quality of Life

PAD has also an impact on patients' quality of life. It is seen that the studies conducted with PAD patients also evaluate the quality of life and health-related quality of life. For example, one study compared 150 patients with PAD and 150 healthy controls. It was concluded that PAD severity with mild, moderate and severe levels was not related to quality of life or perceived stress. However, it was stated that PAD patients had lower quality of life than healthy controls. In addition, participants with type D personality trait reported more negative quality of life. It has been reported that type D personality trait increases the risk of impairment in quality of life and perceived stress, whether the participants have PAD or not

(Aquarius et al. 2005, 996). In parallel with the finding that the quality of life of PAD patients is lower than healthy controls, it is stated that the health-related quality of life of PAD patients and individuals suspected of having PAD has decreased (Reiner et al. 2021, 227). In another study, themes related to quality of life were determined. In this context, 35 themes determined were gathered in 6 main groups. It has been concluded that these groups have symptoms, effect on physical functionality, effect on social functioning, psychological effect, financial impact and care process. It has been stated that these are the main areas that affect the lives of patients living with PAD (Aber et al. 2018, 489). As a result, it is seen that, regardless of the level of having PAD, it negatively affects the quality of life of individuals and this effect focuses on certain themes.

In addition to the effects of PAD on the quality of life of individuals, factors that predict the health-related quality of life of PAD patients were also examined. For example, for the physical functionality of health-related quality of life, the Walking Impairment Questionnaire speed score, history of stumbling, Walking Impairment Questionnaire stair climbing score, activities of daily living associated with bathing, 6 minute walk distance and daily walking cadence were found to be predictors of physical function subscale of health related quality of life scale. In addition, history of stumbling, activities of living related to transferring from bed to a chair and Walking Impairment Questionnaire distance score predicted emotional function subscale of health related quality of life scale. From this, it was concluded that physical and mental sub-dimensions of quality of life were predicted by patient-related physical functioning rather than PAD severity or comorbid conditions. It has been concluded that interventions aimed at improving the health-related quality of life of PAD patients should focus on physical functioning (Gardner et al. 2018, 1126). In conclusion, while physical functionality appears to be a theme in the context of quality of life in PAD patients, it has been concluded that it is the most important predictor of quality of life in this study.

In addition to examining the quality of life in PAD patients, the quality of life of individuals who were intervened for PAD was also examined in studies. For example, in a study, a systematic review was conducted to determine the factors affecting the quality of life of individuals experiencing amputation due to PAD. While 12 studies were included in this review, it was concluded that the ability to walk successfully with a prosthesis had the greatest positive effect on patients' quality of life. It has been stated that being older, being male, longer time after amputation, social support level, and the presence of diabetes are negatively related to quality of life (Davie-Smith et al. 2017, 537). In parallel with this study, which found that prosthesis use and quality of life were related, another study examined prosthesis use and health-related quality of life of PAD patients who experienced amputation. While 98 patients participated in the study, 73 patients completed 1-year follow-up measurements. Compared to the first measurements, it was found that there was an increase in the health-related quality of life of the patients in the measurements after 1 year. It was concluded that 56 of the 73 patients who completed it had prostheses. 23 of the prosthesis users use the prosthesis both inside and outside. It has been concluded that the ability to walk with the prosthesis after amputation is important for the patients' health-related quality of life that they move independently (Torbjörnsson et al. 2020, 1). As a result, the quality of life after amputation was examined in the studies, related factors were examined and it was concluded that the ability to use prosthesis is important for quality of life.

In addition to examining individuals experiencing amputation, individuals with and without amputation have also been compared in studies. For example, a study compared 59 patients with PAD who experienced first major lower leg amputation 2.7 years ago on average and a control group consisting of 118 participants who were matched in terms of age and gender. While health-related quality of life was found to be lower in those who experienced amputation compared to the control group, experienced amputation and control participants reported similar general state of health, life satisfaction and perceived social support. It has been concluded that individuals experiencing amputation have more diseases than the control group. It was stated that half of those who experienced amputation received institutional care and those who received institutional care and those who did not use prosthesis reported more symptoms than those living at home or using prosthesis (Remes et al. 2010, 395). It is concluded that individuals who experience amputation have lower health-related quality of life and more disease than those who do not experience amputation. However, it is seen that there are factors that may be protective in terms of symptoms in those who experience amputation.

There are many different procedures that PAD patients experience as well as amputation. After these procedures, many studies were conducted on the quality of life, psychological health and health-related behaviors of individuals. For example, a study examined the health-related quality of life of PAD patients with percutaneous transluminal angioplasty. Compared to the first measurements of the participants, it was concluded that there was an increase in health-related quality of life in follow-up measurements 1 month and 1 year later (Egberg et al. 2010, 72). In addition to this study in which the quality of life of individuals experiencing percutaneous transluminal angioplasty was examined, another study aimed to examine the quality of life of PAD patients who experienced surgical and/or endovascular revascularization. While 90 patients with PAD participated in the study, measurements were taken before admission and 6 months after discharge. It was concluded that the surgical and / or endovascular revascularization of PAD patients improved their level of movement and usual physical activity, improving their health and improving their quality of life by reducing their pain, discomfort, anxiety and depression. Compared to men, women's quality of life improved more after experiencing revascularization (Staneva et al. 2014). These studies show that PAD patients who undergo these procedures experience positive results in terms of quality of life.

In one study, 711 participants were followed for 5 years after vascular surgery. The effect of smoking cessation on quality of life has been studied. It was concluded that the quality of life of the participants who quit smoking within 3 years after vascular surgery did not increase compared to the participants who continued to smoke. Participants who continue to smoke are more likely to experience deterioration in their quality of life. Although it has been demonstrated that smoking cessation does not make a difference on quality of life, it has been emphasized that smoking cessation should be the main goal, based on the relationships between smoking, complications and mortality in PAD patients (Hoogwegt et al. 2010, 355).

As a result, the quality of life and health-related quality of life of PAD patients were examined in studies. In this context, determining factors are discussed as well as comparison studies. In addition, the quality of life of PAD patients after their treatment has also been examined in studies.

CONCLUSION

PAD is a global problem and in many ways affects how patients live their lives as before. As the mobility of the patients is affected, they can have consequences up to amputation. Not only patients but also caregivers and family members are negatively affected by this disease. It is observed that the patients' quality of life, movements, independence and psychology are negatively affected. It is seen that there are many treatments performed in this sense. Risk factors for PAD have been determined, and a change can be made for risk factors and other treatment methods can be applied. It is observed that studies focus more on the change of risk factors, and it is observed that psychological intervention studies are relatively less. It is observed that the psychology of the patients is also affected and more psychological intervention studies are needed for this disorder, which is expected to increase in the following years. It is predicted that these studies will be beneficial not only for patients but also for family members and caregivers.

REFERENCES

Abaraogu, Ukachukwu Okoroafor, Elochukwu Fortune Ezenwankwo, Philippa Margaret Dall, and Chris Andrew Seenan. "Living a burdensome and demanding life: A qualitative systematic review of the patients experiences of peripheral arterial disease." *PloS one* 13, no. 11 (2018): e0207456.

Aber, Ahmed, Elizabeth Lumley, Patrick Phillips, Helen Buckley Woods, Georgina Jones, and Jonathan Michaels. "Themes that determine quality of life in patients with peripheral arterial disease: a systematic review." *The Patient-Patient-Centered Outcomes Research* 11, no. 5 (2018): 489-502.

Aboyans, Victor, Jean-Baptiste Ricco, Marie-Louise EL Bartelink, Martin Björck, Marianne Brodmann, Tina Cohnert, Jean-Philippe Collet et al. "2017 ESC Guidelines on the Diagnosis and Treatment of Peripheral Arterial Diseases, in collaboration with the European Society for Vascular Surgery (ESVS) Document covering atherosclerotic disease of extracranial carotid and vertebral, mesenteric, renal, upper and lower extremity arteries Endorsed by: the European Stroke Organization (ESO) The Task Force for the Diagnosis and Treatment of Peripheral Arterial Diseases of the European Society of Cardiology (ESC) and of the European Society for Vascular ...." *European heart journal* 39, no. 9 (2018): 763-816.

Al-Delaimy, Wael K., Anwar T. Merchant, Eric B. Rimm, Walter C. Willett, Meir J. Stampfer, and Frank B. Hu. "Effect of type 2 diabetes and its duration on the risk of peripheral arterial disease among men." *The American journal of medicine* 116, no. 4 (2004): 236-240.

American Diabetes Association. "Peripheral arterial disease in people with diabetes." *Diabetes care* 26, no. 12 (2003): 3333-3341.

Aquarius, Annelies E., Johan Denollet, Jaap F. Hamming, Dennis P. Van Berge Henegouwen, and Jolanda De Vries. "Type-D personality and ankle brachial index as predictors of impaired quality of life and depressive symptoms in peripheral arterial disease." *Archives of Surgery* 142, no. 7 (2007): 662-667.

Aquarius, Annelies E., Johan Denollet, Jaap F. Hamming, and Jolanda De Vries. "Role of disease status and type D personality in outcomes in patients with peripheral arterial disease." *The American journal of cardiology* 96, no. 7 (2005): 996-1001.

Aragão, José Aderval, Larissa Gabrielly Ribeiro de Andrade, Osmar Max Gonçalves Neves, Iapunira Catarina Sant'Anna Aragão, Felipe Matheus Sant'Anna Aragão, and Francisco Prado Reis. "Anxiety and depression in patients with peripheral arterial disease admitted to a tertiary hospital." *Journal vascular brasileiro* 18 (2019): 1-11.

Armstrong, Ehrin J., Julie Wu, Gagan D. Singh, David L. Dawson, William C. Pevec, Ezra A. Amsterdam, and John R. Laird. "Smoking cessation is associated with decreased mortality and improved amputation-free survival among patients with symptomatic peripheral artery disease." *Journal of vascular surgery* 60, no. 6 (2014): 1565-1571.

Arseven, Adnan, Jack M. Guralnik, Erin O'Brien, Kiang Liu, and Mary McGrae McDermott. "Peripheral arterial disease and depressed mood in older men and women." *Vascular medicine* 6, no. 4 (2001): 229-234.

Athyros, Vasilios G., Evangelos N. Liberopoulos, Dimitri P. Mikhailidis, Athanasios A. Papageorgiou, Emmanuel S. Ganotakis, Konstantinos Tziomalos, Anna I. Kakafika, Asterios Karagiannis, Stylianos Lambropoulos, and Moses Elisaf. "Association of drinking pattern and alcohol beverage type with the prevalence of metabolic syndrome, diabetes, coronary heart disease, stroke, and peripheral arterial disease in a Mediterranean cohort." *Angiology* 58, no. 6 (2007): 689-697.

Barochiner, Jessica, Lucas S. Aparicio, and Gabriel D. Waisman. "Challenges associated with peripheral arterial disease in women." *Vascular health and risk management* 10 (2014): 115-128.

Batelaan, Neeltje M., Adrie Seldenrijk, Mariska Bot, Anton JLM van Balkom, and Brenda WJH Penninx. "Anxiety and new onset of cardiovascular disease: critical review and meta-analysis." *The British journal of psychiatry* 208, no. 3 (2016): 223-231.

Bell, Steven, Marina Daskalopoulou, Eleni Rapsomaniki, Julie George, Annie Britton, Martin Bobak, Juan P. Casas et al. "Association between clinically recorded alcohol consumption and initial presentation of 12 cardiovascular diseases: population based cohort study using linked health records." *BMJ* 356 (2017): 1-11.

Brostow, Diana P., Megan L. Petrik, Amy J. Starosta, and Stephen W. Waldo. "Depression in patients with peripheral arterial disease: a systematic review." *European Journal of Cardiovascular Nursing* 16, no. 3 (2017): 181-193.

Burton, Nicola W., Zanfina Ademi, Stuart Best, Maria A. Fiatarone Singh, Jason S. Jenkins, Kenny D. Lawson, Anthony S. Leicht et al. "Efficacy of brief behavioral counselling by allied health professionals to promote physical activity in people with peripheral arterial disease (BIPP): study protocol for a multi-center randomized controlled trial." *BMC public health* 16, no. 1 (2016): 1-14.

Camargo, Carlos A., Meir J. Stampfer, Robert J. Glynn, J. Michael Gaziano, JoAnn E. Manson, Samuel Z. Goldhaber, and Charles H. Hennekens. "Prospective study of moderate alcohol consumption and risk of peripheral arterial disease in US male physicians." *Circulation* 95, no. 3 (1997): 577-580.

Chi, Yung-Wei, and Michael R. Jaff. "Optimal risk factor modification and medical management of the patient with peripheral arterial disease." *Catheterization and Cardiovascular Interventions* 71, no. 4 (2008): 475-489.

Columbo, Jesse A., David H. Stone, Philip P. Goodney, Brian W. Nolan, Jennifer A. Stableford, Benjamin S. Brooke, Richard J. Powell, and Christine T. Finn. "The prevalence and regional variation of major depressive disorder among patients with peripheral arterial disease in the Medicare population." *Vascular and endovascular surgery* 50, no. 4 (2016): 235-240.

Conen, David, Brendan M. Everett, Tobias Kurth, Mark A. Creager, Julie E. Buring, Paul M. Ridker, and Aruna D. Pradhan. "Smoking, smoking cessation, and risk for symptomatic peripheral artery disease in women: a cohort study." *Annals of internal medicine* 154, no. 11 (2011): 719-726.

Criqui, Michael H., Julie O. Denenberg, Robert D. Langer, and Arnost Fronek. "The epidemiology of peripheral arterial disease: importance of identifying the population at risk." *Vascular Medicine* 2, no. 3 (1997): 221-226.

Cunningham, M. A., Vivien Swanson, R. J. Holdsworth, and R. E. O'Carroll. "Late effects of a brief psychological intervention in patients with intermittent claudication in a randomized clinical trial." *British Journal of Surgery* 100, no. 6 (2013): 756-760.

Cunningham, M. A., Vivien Swanson, R. E. O'Caroll, and R. J. Holdsworth. "Randomized clinical trial of a brief psychological intervention to increase walking in patients with intermittent claudication." *British Journal of Surgery* 99, no. 6 (2012): 854-854.

Daskalopoulou, Marina, Julie George, Kate Walters, David P. Osborn, G. David Batty, Dimitris Stogiannis, Eleni Rapsomaniki et al. "Depression as a risk factor for the initial presentation of twelve cardiac, cerebrovascular, and peripheral arterial diseases: data linkage study of 1.9 million women and men." *PloS one* 11, no. 4 (2016): e0153838.

Davie-Smith, Fiona, Elaine Coulter, Brian Kennon, Sally Wyke, and Lorna Paul. "Factors influencing quality of life following lower limb amputation for peripheral arterial occlusive disease: A systematic review of the literature." *Prosthetics and orthotics international* 41, no. 6 (2017): 537-547.

Desormais, I., Aboyans, V., Guerchet, M., Ndamba-Bandzouzi, B., Mbelesso, P., Magne, J., ... & Preux, P. M. (2019). Body mass index and peripheral arterial disease, a U-shaped relationship in elderly African population–the EPIDEMCA study. *Vasa, 49,* 50-56.

Devrome, A. N., Aggarwal, S., McMurtry, M. S., Southern, D., Hauer, T., Lamb, B., ... & Martin, B. J. (2019). Cardiac rehabilitation in people with peripheral arterial disease: A higher risk population that benefits from completion. *International journal of cardiology, 285,* 108-114.

Diaconescu, Liliana Veronica, and Ion Diaconescu. "Protective Factors Against Depression In Patients With Peripheral Arterial Disease With Critical Limb Ischemia." *Romanian Medical Journal* 64, no. 4 (2017): 296-299.

Donnan, Peter T., Marjory Thomson, F. G. Fowkes, Robin J. Prescott, and Edward Housley. "Diet as a risk factor for peripheral arterial disease in the general population: the Edinburgh Artery Study." *The American journal of clinical nutrition* 57, no. 6 (1993): 917-921.

Egberg, Louise, Sissel Andreassen, and Anne-Cathrine Mattiasson. "Living a demanding life–spouses' experiences of living with a person suffering from intermittent claudication." *Journal of advanced nursing* 69, no. 3 (2013): 610-618.

Egberg, Louise, Anne-Cathrine Mattiasson, Karl-Gösta Ljungström, and Johan Styrud. "Health-related quality of life in patients with peripheral arterial disease undergoing percutaneous transluminal angioplasty: a prospective one-year follow-up." *Journal of Vascular Nursing* 28, no. 2 (2010): 72-77.

Elfghi, Marah, Fionnuala Jordan, Denise Dunne, Irene Gibson, Jennifer Jones, Gerard Flaherty, Sherif Sultan, and Wael Tawfick. "The effect of lifestyle and risk factor modification on occlusive peripheral arterial disease outcomes: standard healthcare vs structured programme—for a randomised controlled trial protocol." *Trials* 22, no. 1 (2021): 1-10.

Faglia, Ezio. "Characteristics of peripheral arterial disease and its relevance to the diabetic population." *The international journal of lower extremity wounds* 10, no. 3 (2011): 152-166.

Fakhry, Farzin, Koen M. van de Luijtgaarden, Leon Bax, P. Ted den Hoed, MG Myriam Hunink, Ellen V. Rouwet, and Sandra Spronk. "Supervised walking therapy in patients with intermittent claudication." *Journal of Vascular Surgery* 56, no. 4 (2012): 1132-1142.

Fowkes, F. G. R. "The measurement of atherosclerotic peripheral arterial disease in epidemiological surveys." *International journal of epidemiology* 17, no. 2 (1988): 248-254.

Fowler, Bess, Konrad Jamrozik, Paul Norman, and Yvonne Allen. "Prevalence of peripheral arterial disease: persistence of excess risk in former smokers." *Australian and New Zealand journal of public health* 26, no. 3 (2007): 219-224.

Galloway, S., N. Bubela, A. McKibbon, D. Rebeyka, and M. Saxe-Braithwaite. "Symptom distress, anxiety, depression, and discharge information needs after peripheral arterial bypass." *Journal of Vascular Nursing* 13, no. 2 (1995): 35-40.

Gardner, Andrew W., Polly S. Montgomery, Ming Wang, and Cong Xu. "Predictors of health-related quality of life in patients with symptomatic peripheral artery disease." *Journal of vascular surgery* 68, no. 4 (2018): 1126-1134.

Garnefski, N., M. Grol, V. Kraaij, and J. F. Hamming. "Cognitive coping and goal adjustment in people with Peripheral Arterial Disease: Relationships with depressive symptoms." *Patient Education and Counseling* 76, no. 1 (2009): 132-137.

Garnefski, N., V. Kraaij, E. Wijers, and J. Hamming. "Effects of a cognitive-behavioral self-help program on depressed mood for people with peripheral arterial disease." *Journal of clinical psychology in medical settings* 20, no. 2 (2013): 186-191.

Grenon, S. Marlene, Beth E. Cohen, Kim Smolderen, Eric Vittinghoff, Mary A. Whooley, and Jade Hiramoto. "Peripheral arterial disease, gender, and depression in the Heart and Soul Study." *Journal of vascular surgery* 60, no. 2 (2014): 396-403.

Harwood, Amy-Elizabeth, George E. Smith, Thomas Cayton, Edward Broadbent, and Ian C. Chetter. "A systematic review of the uptake and adherence rates to supervised exercise programs in patients with intermittent claudication." *Annals of vascular surgery* 34 (2016): 280-289.

He, Yao, Yong Jiang, Jie Wang, Li Fan, XiaoYing Li, and Frank B. Hu. "Prevalence of peripheral arterial disease and its association with smoking in a population-based study in Beijing, China." *Journal of vascular surgery* 44, no. 2 (2006): 333-338.

He, Yao, Tai Hing Lam, Bin Jiang, Jie Wang, Xiaoyong Sai, Li Fan, Xiaoying Li, Yinhe Qin, and Frank B. Hu. "Passive smoking and risk of peripheral arterial disease and ischemic stroke in Chinese women who never smoked." *Circulation* 118, no. 15 (2008): 1535-1540.

Heffron, S. P., Dwivedi, A., Rockman, C. B., Xia, Y., Guo, Y., Zhong, J., & Berger, J. S. (2020). Body mass index and peripheral artery disease. *Atherosclerosis*, *292*, 31-36.

Heffron, Sean P., Caron B. Rockman, Eugenia Gianos, Yu Guo, and Jeffrey S. Berger. "Greater frequency of nut consumption is associated with lower prevalence of peripheral arterial disease." *Preventive medicine* 72 (2015): 15-18.

Hennrikus, Deborah, Anne M. Joseph, Harry A. Lando, Sue Duval, Laurie Ukestad, Molly Kodl, and Alan T. Hirsch. "Effectiveness of a smoking cessation program for peripheral artery disease patients: a randomized controlled trial." *Journal of the American College of Cardiology* 56, no. 25 (2010): 2105-2112.

Hiatt, William R. "Medical treatment of peripheral arterial disease and claudication." *New England Journal of Medicine* 344, no. 21 (2001): 1608-1621.

Hobbs, S. D., and A. W. Bradbury. "Smoking cessation strategies in patients with peripheral arterial disease: an evidence-based approach." *European journal of vascular and endovascular surgery* 26, no. 4 (2003): 341-347.

Hoogwegt, M. T., S. E. Hoeks, Susanne S. Pedersen, WJM Scholte op Reimer, Y. R. B. M. van Gestel, H. J. M. Verhagen, and Don Poldermans. "Smoking cessation has no influence on quality of life in patients with peripheral arterial disease 5 years post-vascular surgery." *European Journal of Vascular and Endovascular Surgery* 40, no. 3 (2010): 355-362.

Housley, E., G. C. Leng, P. T. Donnan, and F. G. Fowkes. "Physical activity and risk of peripheral arterial disease in the general population: Edinburgh Artery Study." *Journal of Epidemiology & Community Health* 47, no. 6 (1993): 475-480.

Huang, Jin-Yuan, Wei-Kung Chen, Cheng-Li Lin, Ching-Yuan Lai, Chia-Hung Kao, and Tse-Yen Yang. "Increased risk of peripheral arterial disease in patients with alcohol intoxication: A population-based retrospective cohort study." *Alcohol* 65 (2017): 25-30.

Huang, Ya, Min Xu, Lan Xie, Tiange Wang, Xiaolin Huang, Xiaofei Lv, Ying Chen et al. "Obesity and peripheral arterial disease: a Mendelian randomization analysis." *Atherosclerosis* 247 (2016): 218-224.

Hung, Hsin-Chia, Anwar Merchant, Walter Willett, Alberto Ascherio, Bernard A. Rosner, Eric Rimm, and Kaumudi J. Joshipura. "The association between fruit and vegetable consumption and peripheral arterial disease." *Epidemiology* (2003): 659-665.

James, Spencer L., Degu Abate, Kalkidan Hassen Abate, Solomon M. Abay, Cristiana Abbafati, Nooshin Abbasi, Hedayat Abbastabar et al. "Global, regional, and national incidence, prevalence, and years lived with disability for 354 diseases and injuries for 195 countries and territories, 1990–2017: a systematic analysis for the Global Burden of Disease Study 2017." *The Lancet* 392, no. 10159 (2018): 1789-1858.

Johnstone, C. C. (2004). Living with peripheral vascular disease: patients and their carers. *Nursing times*, *100*(39), 36-39.

Jude, E. B., I. Eleftheriadou, and N. Tentolouris. "Peripheral arterial disease in diabetes—a review." *Diabetic medicine* 27, no. 1 (2010): 4-14.

Kolossváry, E., Tamás Ferenci, T. Kováts, Levente Kovács, Z. Járai, Gábor Menyhei, and Katalin Farkas. "Trends in major lower limb amputation related to peripheral arterial disease in Hungary: a nationwide study (2004–2012)." *European Journal of Vascular and Endovascular Surgery* 50, no. 1 (2015): 78-85.

Kröger, Knut, Andreas Stang, Jana Kondratieva, Susanne Moebus, Eva Beck, Axel Schmermund, Stefan Möhlenkamp et al. "Prevalence of peripheral arterial disease–results of the Heinz Nixdorf recall study." *European journal of epidemiology* 21, no. 4 (2006): 279-285.

Kumar, Anjana M., Angela K. Lyden, Noelle E. Carlozzi, Ananda Sen, Caroline R. Richardson, and Elizabeth A. Jackson. "The Physical Activity Daily (PAD) Trial: The rationale and design of a randomized controlled trial evaluating an internet walking program to improve maximal walking distance among patients with peripheral arterial disease." *Contemporary clinical trials* 67 (2018): 23-30.

Lamberti, Nicola, Sofia Straudi, Roberto Manfredini, Alfredo De Giorgi, Vincenzo Gasbarro, Paolo Zamboni, and Fabio Manfredini. "Don't stop walking: the in-home rehabilitation program for peripheral artery disease patients during the COVID-19 pandemic." *Internal and emergency medicine* (2021): 1-9.

Lu, L., D. F. Mackay, and J. P. Pell. "Meta-analysis of the association between cigarette smoking and peripheral arterial disease." *Heart* 100, no. 5 (2014): 414-423.

Marso, Steven P., and William R. Hiatt. "Peripheral arterial disease in patients with diabetes." *Journal of the American College of Cardiology* 47, no. 5 (2006): 921-929.

Mattioli, Anna Vittoria, Francesca Coppi, Mario Migaldi, P. Scicchitano, M. M. Ciccone, and Alberto Farinetti. "Relationship between Mediterranean diet and asymptomatic peripheral arterial disease in a population of pre-menopausal women." *Nutrition, Metabolism and Cardiovascular Diseases* 27, no. 11 (2017): 985-990.

McCallum, Mary, Benjamin Cooper, Samantha Matson, Bryce Renwick, and Sarah Jane Messeder. "Improving health behaviors in patients with peripheral arterial disease–A pilot study of supported self-management." *Journal of Vascular Nursing* (2020).

McDermott, Mary McGrae, Philip Greenland, Jack M. Guralnik, Kiang Liu, Michael H. Criqui, William H. Pearce, Cheeling Chan et al. "Depressive symptoms and lower extremity functioning in men and women with peripheral arterial disease." *Journal of general internal medicine* 18, no. 6 (2003): 461-467.

McDermott, M. M., Guralnik, J. M., Criqui, M. H., Ferrucci, L., Zhao, L., Liu, K., ... & Rejeski, W. J. (2014). Home-based walking exercise in peripheral artery disease: 12-month follow-up of the GOALS randomized trial. *Journal of the American Heart Association*, *3*(3), e000711.

McDermott, M. M., Guralnik, J. M., Criqui, M. H., Ferrucci, L., Liu, K., Spring, B., ... & Rejeski, W. J. (2015). Unsupervised exercise and mobility loss in peripheral artery disease: a randomized controlled trial. *Journal of the American Heart Association*, *4*(5), e001659.

McDermott, Mary M., William B. Applegate, Denise E. Bonds, Thomas W. Buford, Timothy Church, Mark A. Espeland, Thomas M. Gill et al. "Ankle brachial index values, leg symptoms, and functional performance among community-dwelling older men and women in the lifestyle interventions and independence for elders study." *Journal of the American Heart Association* 2, no. 6 (2013): e000257.

McDermott, Mary M., Susan Tiukinhoy, Philip Greenland, Kiang Liu, William H. Pearce, Jack M. Guralnik, Shay Unterreiner, Ty J. Gluckman, Michael H. Criqui, and Luigi Ferrucci. *A pilot exercise intervention to improve lower extremity functioning in peripheral arterial disease unaccompanied by intermittent claudication.* (2004): 187-196.

Meijer, Wouter T., Diederick E. Grobbee, MG Myriam Hunink, Albert Hofman, and Arno W. Hoes. "Determinants of peripheral arterial disease in the elderly: the Rotterdam study." *Archives of internal medicine* 160, no. 19 (2000): 2934-2938.

Merchant, Anwar T., Frank B. Hu, Donna Spiegelman, Walter C. Willett, Eric B. Rimm, and Alberto Ascherio. "Dietary fiber reduces peripheral arterial disease risk in men." *The Journal of nutrition* 133, no. 11 (2003): 3658-3663.

Montgomery, Polly S., and Andrew W. Gardner. "The clinical utility of a six-minute walk test in peripheral arterial occlusive disease patients." *Journal of the American Geriatrics Society* 46, no. 6 (1998): 706-711.

Mukherjee, D., and J. S. Yadav. "Update on peripheral vascular diseases: from smoking cessation to stenting." *Cleveland Clinic journal of medicine* 68, no. 8 (2001): 723-733.

Murabito, Joanne M., Jane C. Evans, Kenneth Nieto, Martin G. Larson, Daniel Levy, and Peter WF Wilson. "Prevalence and clinical correlates of peripheral arterial disease in the Framingham Offspring Study." *American heart journal* 143, no. 6 (2002): 961-965.

Newhall, Karina, Bjoern Suckow, Emily Spangler, Benjamin S. Brooke, Andres Schanzer, Tze-Woei Tan, Mary Burnette, Maria Orlando Edelen, Alik Farber, and Philip Goodney. "Impact and duration of brief surgeon-delivered smoking cessation advice on attitudes regarding nicotine dependence and tobacco harms for patients with peripheral arterial disease." *Annals of vascular surgery* 38 (2017): 113-121.

Ogilvie, Rachel P., Pamela L. Lutsey, Gerardo Heiss, Aaron R. Folsom, and Lyn M. Steffen. "Dietary intake and peripheral arterial disease incidence in middle-aged adults: the Atherosclerosis Risk in Communities (ARIC) Study." *The American journal of clinical nutrition* 105, no. 3 (2017): 651-659.

Parvar, Saman L., Robert Fitridge, Joseph Dawson, and Stephen J. Nicholls. "Medical and lifestyle management of peripheral arterial disease." *Journal of vascular surgery* 68, no. 5 (2018): 1595-1606.

Pilz, Magdalena, Elisabeth Kandioler-Honetz, Alfa Wenkstetten-Holub, Waltraud Doerrscheidt, Rudolf Mueller, and Robert Wolfgang Kurz. "Evaluation of 6-and 12-month supervised exercise training on strength and endurance parameters in patients with peripheral arterial disease." *Wiener Klinische Wochenschrift* 126, no. 11 (2014): 383-389.

Powell, Janet T., Richard J. Edwards, Phillip C. Worrell, Peter J. Franks, Roger M. Greenhalgh, and Neil R. Poulter. "Risk factors associated with the development of peripheral arterial disease in smokers: a case-control study." *Atherosclerosis* 129, no. 1 (1997): 41-48.

Price, JF1, P. I. Mowbray, A. J. Lee, A. Rumley, G. D. O. Lowe, and F. G. R. Fowkes. "Relationship between smoking and cardiovascular risk factors in the development of peripheral arterial disease and coronary artery disease; Edinburgh Artery Study: Edinburgh Artery Study." *European heart journal* 20, no. 5 (1999): 344-353.

Ragazzo, Luciana, Pedro Puech-Leao, Nelson Wolosker, Nelson de Luccia, Glauco Saes, Raphael M. Ritti-Dias, Gabriel Grizzo Cucato, Debora Yumi Ferreira Kamikava, and Antonio Eduardo Zerati. "Symptoms of anxiety and depression and their relationship with barriers to physical activity in patients with intermittent claudication." *Clinics* 76, no. 76 (2021): e1802.

Ramirez, Joel L., Laura M. Drudi, and S. Marlene Grenon. "Review of biologic and behavioral risk factors linking depression and peripheral artery disease." *Vascular Medicine* 23, no. 5 (2018): 478-488.

Reiner, Željko, Johan De Sutter, Lars Ryden, Erkin Mirrakhimov, Nana Pogosova, Marina Dolzhenko, Zlatko Fras, Kornelia Kotseva, David Wood, and Dirk De Bacquer. "Peripheral arterial disease and intermittent claudication in coronary heart disease patients." *International Journal of Cardiology* 322 (2021): 227-232.

Rejeski, W. Jack, Bonnie Spring, Kathryn Domanchuk, Huimin Tao, Lu Tian, Lihui Zhao, and Mary M. McDermott. "A group-mediated, home-based physical activity intervention for patients with peripheral artery disease: effects on social and psychological function." *Journal of translational medicine* 12, no. 1 (2014): 1-8.

Remes, Leena, Raimo Isoaho, Tero Vahlberg, Matti Viitanen, Markku Koskenvuo, and Päivi Rautava. "Quality of life three years after major lower extremity amputation due to peripheral arterial disease." *Aging clinical and experimental research* 22, no. 5 (2010): 395-405.

Ruiz-Canela, Miguel, Ramón Estruch, Dolores Corella, Jordi Salas-Salvadó, and Miguel A. Martínez-González. "Association of Mediterranean diet with peripheral artery disease: the PREDIMED randomized trial." *Jama* 311, no. 4 (2014): 415-417.

Ruo, Bernice, Kiang Liu, Lu Tian, Jin Tan, Luigi Ferrucci, Jack M. Guralnik, and Mary M. McDermott. "Persistent depressive symptoms and functional decline among patients with peripheral arterial disease." *Psychosomatic medicine* 69, no. 5 (2007): 415-424.

Sampson, Uchechukwu KA, F. Gerald R. Fowkes, Mary M. McDermott, Michael H. Criqui, Victor Aboyans, Paul E. Norman, Mohammad H. Forouzanfar et al. "Global and regional burden of death and disability from peripheral artery disease: 21 world regions, 1990 to 2010." *Global heart* 9, no. 1 (2014): 145-158.

Smolderen, Kim GE, Annelies E. Aquarius, Jolanda de Vries, Otto RF Smith, Jaap F. Hamming, and Johan Denollet. "Depressive symptoms in peripheral arterial disease: a follow-up study on prevalence, stability, and risk factors." *Journal of affective disorders* 110, no. 1-2 (2008): 27-35.

Smolderen, Kim G., Sanne E. Hoeks, Susanne S. Pedersen, Ron T. van Domburg, Inge I. de Liefde, and Don Poldermans. "Lower-leg symptoms in peripheral arterial disease are associated with anxiety, depression, and anhedonia." *Vascular Medicine* 14, no. 4 (2009): 297-304.

Song, Peige, Diana Rudan, Yajie Zhu, Freya JI Fowkes, Kazem Rahimi, F. Gerald R. Fowkes, and Igor Rudan. "Global, regional, and national prevalence and risk factors for peripheral artery disease in 2015: an updated systematic review and analysis." *The Lancet Global Health* 7, no. 8 (2019): e1020-e1030.

Staneva, M., Tz Tzvetanov, B. Minkova, P. Antova, and V. Chervenkoff. "Quality of life of patients with lower extremity peripheral arterial disease." *Scripta Scientifica Medica* 46, no. 1 (2014).

Thomas, Merrill, Donna M. Buchanan, Krishna K. Patel, Kensey Gosch, and Kim Smolderen. "Mental health concerns in patients presenting with new or an exacerbation of peripheral arterial disease symptoms: insights from the international portrait registry." *Journal of the American College of Cardiology* 71, no. 11S (2018): A2040-A2040.

Thomas, Merrill, Krishna K. Patel, Kensey Gosch, Clementine Labrosciano, Carlos Mena-Hurtado, Robert Fitridge, John A. Spertus, and Kim G. Smolderen. "Mental health concerns in patients with symptomatic peripheral artery disease: Insights from the PORTRAIT registry." *Journal of psychosomatic research* 131 (2020): 109963.

Torbjörnsson, Eva, Carin Ottosson, Lena Blomgren, Lennart Boström, and Ann-Mari Fagerdahl. "The patient's experience of amputation due to peripheral arterial disease." *Journal of Vascular Nursing* 35, no. 2 (2017): 57-63.

Torbjörnsson, Eva, Carin Ottosson, Lennart Boström, Lena Blomgren, Jonas Malmstedt, and Ann-Mari Fagerdahl. "Health-related quality of life and prosthesis use among patients amputated due to peripheral arterial disease–a one-year follow-up." *Disability and Rehabilitation* (2020): 1-9.

Tóth-Vajna, Gergely, Zsombor Tóth-Vajna, Piroska Balog, and Barna Konkolÿ Thege. "Depressive symptomatology and personality traits in patients with symptomatic and asymptomatic peripheral arterial disease." *BMC cardiovascular disorders* 20, no. 1 (2020): 1-8.

Turner, Aaron P., Rhonda M. Williams, Daniel C. Norvell, Alison W. Henderson, Kevin N. Hakimi, Donna Jo Blake, and Joseph M. Czerniecki. "Prevalence and 1-year course of alcohol misuse and smoking in persons with lower extremity amputation as a result of peripheral arterial disease." *American journal of physical medicine & rehabilitation* 93, no. 6 (2014): 493-502.

Unkart, Jonathan T., Matthew A. Allison, Humberto Parada Jr, Michael H. Criqui, Qibin Qi, Keith M. Diaz, Jordan A. Carlson et al. "Sedentary time and peripheral artery disease: the Hispanic community health study/study of Latinos." *American heart journal* 222 (2020): 208-219.

Verma, Anil, Amit Prasad, Ghasan H. Elkadi, and Yung-Wei Chi. "Peripheral arterial disease: evaluation, risk factor modification, and medical management." *Journal of Clinical Outcomes Management* 18, no. 2 (2011): 34-47.

Vliegenthart, Rozemarijn, Johanna M. Geleijnse, Albert Hofman, Wouter T. Meijer, Frank JA van Rooij, Diederick E. Grobbee, and Jacqueline CM Witteman. "Alcohol consumption and risk of peripheral arterial disease: the Rotterdam study." *American journal of epidemiology* 155, no. 4 (2002): 332-338.

Wann-Hansson, Christine, I. R. Hallberg, Rosemarie Klevsgård, and Edith Andersson. "Patients' experiences of living with peripheral arterial disease awaiting intervention: a qualitative study." *International Journal of Nursing Studies* 42, no. 8 (2005): 851-862.

Wann-Hansson, Christine, Ingalill Rahm Hallberg, Rosemarie Klevsgård, and Edith Andersson. "The long-term experience of living with peripheral arterial disease and the recovery following revascularisation: A qualitative study." *International journal of nursing studies* 45, no. 4 (2008): 552-561.

Wattanakit, Keattiyoat, Janice E. Williams, Pamela J. Schreiner, Alan T. Hirsch, and Aaron R. Folsom. "Association of anger proneness, depression and low social support with peripheral arterial disease: the Atherosclerosis Risk in Communities Study." *Vascular medicine* 10, no. 3 (2005): 199-206.

Willigendael, Edith M., Joep AW Teijink, Marie-Louise Bartelink, Barthold W. Kuiken, Jelis Boiten, Frans L. Moll, Harry R. Büller, and Martin H. Prins. "Influence of smoking on incidence and prevalence of peripheral arterial disease." *Journal of vascular surgery* 40, no. 6 (2004): 1158-1165.

Wong, Samuel YS, Jean Woo, Athena WL Hong, Jason CS Leung, and Ping C. Leung. "Clinically relevant depressive symptoms and peripheral arterial disease in elderly men and women. Results from a large cohort study in Southern China." *Journal of psychosomatic research* 63, no. 5 (2007): 471-476.

Wongkongkam, Kessiri, Orapan Thosingha, Chanean Ruangsetakit, Kewwalee Phuntep, and Sununta Tonklai. "Psychological factors associated with functional recovery among patients with a peripheral arterial disease after lower extremity bypass." *Journal of Vascular Nursing* 37, no. 1 (2019): 3-10.

In: Peripheral Artery Disease
Editor: Jeremy D. Parks

ISBN: 978-1-53619-968-0
© 2021 Nova Science Publishers, Inc.

Chapter 2

DIABETES MANAGEMENT IN PERIPHERAL ARTERY DISEASE PATIENTS

Deniz Dönmez Evinç[1],*, MD and Nilgün Özçakar[2], MD
[1]Milas Provincial Health Directorate, Mugla, Turkey
[2]Department of Family Medicine, Faculty of Medicine,
Dokuz Eylul University, İzmir, Turkey

ABSTRACT

Diabetes, a serious threat for global health together with peripheral artery disease, became a burden for both patients and the health care systems for their social and economic consequences. Each of them is a predictor for the other, and even worsen the prognosis of the patient if they are present at the same time. As a coincidence both group of patients are unaware of their health status, which can progress towards a much serious problem ending with limb loss. The primary care physicians are important for the awareness of patients having diabetes and peripheral artery disease for their increased risk of comorbidity and complications that need follow up for appropriate diagnosis, treatment and referral when needed. In addition, it is important to keep in contact with these patients

---
* Corresponding Author's E-mail: drdeniz78@hotmail.com.

for their life style changes; nutritional behaviors, physical activities and exercise training, blood sugar monitoring and applying medications, risk reduction, problem solving abilities and need for seeking medical care. Often a successful diabetes education, will give the patients a real role in many dietary and lifestyle modifications thus improve self-care significantly, with the support of healthcare professionals, which gives them self-confidence that reduces the mortality and morbidity as well as health care costs and improves the health care quality of life.

Keywords: diabetes, peripheral artery disease, primary care, general practice, patient education, life style changes

INTRODUCTION

Diabetes Mellitus (DM), a silent killer, is a serious threat for global health with half a billion people living with the disease, and is predicted to reach 578 million in 2030 and 700 million in 2045 if urgent prevention strategies are not implemented worldwide. As a chronic disease, diabetes has a serious impact on the lives and well-being of individuals and families all over the world and is among the top 10 causes of death in adults in the society. It is important to encourage diabetes prevention and to encourage improvements in the care of everyone living with diabetes. Despite the increase in prevalence, primary care physicians (PCPs) can contribute to the survival of people with diabetes through early diagnosis, improved diabetes management and, consequently, a reduction in premature death rates. In the 21st century, peripheral artery disease (PAD) has become a global problem as well as diabetes [1, 2]. Both diseases are shown to be each other's predictor and it is true that they worsen each other if both are present at the same time. The governments, non-governmental organizations and private sectors must urgently assess social and economic consequences mostly and especially for the prevention and treatment strategies. Not just PAD but also other serious and life-threatening complications increase the need of medical care, frequent hospital admissions, adding on diabetic patients & their family serious cause of stress and impairs the quality of life seriously. PAD also tends to progress faster and lead to worse outcomes in diabetic patients. It should be noted that therapeutic regimens other than glycemic control strategies may have differential effects on the progression of PAD. Blood pressure medications, lipid-lowering medications, antiplatelet therapy, exercise conditioning, and smoking cessation proposed as potentially viable therapies to reduce the progression of PAD. It should be kept in mind that therapeutic regimens other than glycemic control strategies may have different effects on the progression of PAD [3, 4].

Lower extremity peripheral artery disease is the third leading cause of atherosclerotic cardiovascular morbidity, following coronary artery disease and stroke. Peripheral artery disease is a critical manifestation of atherosclerosis, which is associated with an increased risk of cardiovascular mortality [5]. In both high-income countries and low and middle-income countries the prevalence of peripheral artery disease increases with age; at the age of 60 it is affecting 12% to 20% of Americans and at the age 85 it is up to 50%. The prevalence of PAD is higher among non-Hispanic blacks, and it is more common in smokers, people with low kidney function, and among individuals reporting a history of cardiovascular disease (CVD - coronary heart disease, congestive heart failure, or stroke). More than half of the individuals with PAD reported the presence of hypercholesterolemia, similarly, over 70% had hypertension, one third had diabetes, and almost all of these people are still smoking. Almost all of them had at least one of these CVD risk factors, and those with two or more risk factors are stated to be 70%. One in 3 people with PAD say they have CVD (coronary heart disease, congestive heart failure and / or stroke) [6]. As mentioned in the articles between the years 2000 to 2010 the prevalence increased by 23.5% and became a global health problem that must be studied multidisciplinary. In addition to age, race, smoking, hypertension, and lipids are the other important risk factors that effects the prevalence of PAD. From a 1.5-fold increase with one risk factor with each additional risk factor, provides a 10-fold increase in PAD risk. Among the known risk factors, the majority of individuals with PAD have one or more cardiovascular disease risk factors that should be targeted for treatment [6]. There is also evidence that biomarkers are indicative of inflammation and/or coagulation, such as C-reactive protein (CRP), D-dimer, fibrinogen, and they may be associated with increased PAD risk and/or worse outcomes [5]. Major amputations are mostly caused by infrapopliteal arterial involvement, and there is a higher risk for DM patients. Among PAD patients, the diabetic ones have the worse arterial disease and a poorer outcome compared to nondiabetic patients. Diabetic patients with PAD also had higher mortality and died at a younger age than nondiabetic patients [7].

DIABETES AND PAD TOGETHER, CLINICAL AND ECONOMIC EFFECTS

Diabetes mellitus is the strongest risk factor for peripheral artery disease, after smoking [8]. DM is present in 20% to 30% of patients with PAD and patients with DM have a risk of 2-4 fold for developing PAD. PAD is especially common among patients with DM, with a threefold increased risk compared with the general population. There are associations between traditional (such as hypertension, high cholesterol, diabetes, and smoking) and non-traditional (inflammatory biomarkers such as CRP, D-dimer, and fibrinogen or altered calcium-phosphorus metabolism, homocysteine metabolism, lipoprotein(a) metabolism, and alterations in inflammatory and coagulation pathways) risk factors for PAD and their effect occurs over time in the lower extremities in patients with DM. PAD also tends to progress faster and lead to worse outcomes in DM patients. Moreover, PAD is known to increase the risk of functional limitation, leg revascularization, and amputation. Studies have found that higher baseline pulse pressure; ABI (Ankle Brachial Index) and HbA1c are positively associated with the risk of PAD [5, 9]. These patients also have greater functional impairment due to PAD in terms of shorter walking velocities and distance and greater rates of cardiovascular events compared with those having PAD but not DM. Among patients with diabetes, known cardiovascular risk factors are the main predictors of PAD cases.

Moreover, the prevalence of "traditional" cardiovascular disease risk factors such as hypertension, high cholesterol, diabetes, and smoking was high among persons with PAD. With nearly 95% of persons with prevalent PAD having at least one of these risk factors. Studies have shown that diabetes increases the incidence of limb ischemia four times in patients with PAD. In addition, it has been reported that in diabetic patients with critical limb ischemia, 50% will develop critical limb ischemia in the contralateral leg within 5 years. According to the American Diabetes Association (ADA) consensus, ABI screening recommendations should be included in clinical practice for the following reasons [9].

First of all, an abnormal ABI is strongly associated with an increased risk for coronary heart disease mortality and morbidity. Besides, if PAD is determined, an aggressive secondary prevention medical strategy should be implemented. On the other hand, PAD is underdiagnosed in primary care and this is an important obstacle to the best secondary prevention of ischemic cardiovascular disease. The National Cholesterol Education Program / Adult Treatment Panel III guidelines classify diabetes as a coronary heart disease equivalent and recommend a targeted low-density lipoprotein (LDL) cholesterol level of 100 mg / dl. The latest update to these guidelines recommends a target LDL level of 70 mg / dl for very high-risk patients [10-12].

The diagnostic criteria for diabetes summarized as below;

Table 1. Diagnostic criteria [13]

	FPG	PG in OGTT	A1C
Normal	<100 mg/dL or 5.5 mmol/L	<140 mg/dL or 7.8 mmol/L	<5.7% or 39 mmol/mol
Pre-Diabetes	≥100 mg/dL or 5.5 mmol/L	≥140 mg/dL or 7.8 mmol/L	≥5.7% or 39 mmol/mol
Diabetes	≥126 mg/dL or 7.0 mmol/L	≥200 mg/dL or 11.1 mmol/L	≥6.5% or 48 mmol/mol

FPG: Fasting Plasma Glucose.
PG: (Plasma Glucose) in OGTT: (Oral Glucose Tolerance Test).
A1C: Hemoglobin A1c.

As we mentioned above the dysglycemia types, IFG (Impaired Fasting Glucose) and IGT (Impaired Glucose Tolerance) can be called as the gray area, not diabetic nor normal. They can be converted to normoglycemia with easy and simple interventions of life style changes. Moreover, with adoption to the lifestyle changes, long-term studies have shown that the risk of this progression—from pre-diabetes to diabetes—can be lowered for an extended period of 10 years. Raising awareness and risk stratification of individuals with prediabetes can help doctors understand potential interventions that can help reduce the percentage of patients who will develop diabetes. It is stated that one third of individuals with prediabetes can develop diabetes within 4 years if left untreated, and the percentage of these prediabetic patients who develop diabetes can be reduced to one fifth with lifestyle intervention. Interventions for identifying prediabetic individuals is crucial for our efforts to make healthcare more cost-effective, and save lives preventing diseases. Recent evidence suggests that it is possible to prevent progression of prediabetes to diabetes and to convert prediabetes to a normal glucose level. In addition, prediabetes and diabetes complications can only be prevented by achieving a normal glucose pattern. Studies show that the difference in the direct and indirect costs of caring for a patient with prediabetes and a patient with diabetes can be as much as $ 7000 per year [14]. Pre-diabetes, is a critical phase, since the condition is reversible and could serve as a potential route to combat diabetes. Prediabetes do not increase the risk for microvascular disease as seen in diabetes, the main risk in this condition is the development of diabetes and CVD which makes it important to act before facing the major morbidities. It should not be forgotten that the primary purpose of lifestyle interventions in this regard is to prevent diabetes and its complications by targeting obesity and physical inactivity [15]. For individuals without diabetes, fasting blood glucose concentration is modestly and non-linearly associated with risk of vascular disease [16]. The importance of FPG levels should not be forgotten for preventive interventions. Rising rates of obesity around the world will likely increase the absolute risk for diabetes and vascular disease.

Another emerging fact about PAD is the increasing healthcare cost. The healthcare cost of PAD-related care is having great importance as the effected population increase every year. All over the world, the economic burden of atherothrombotic diseases is high and it is expected to increase further with the increase in the life span with this disease as population aging. The PCPs have a key role for preventive care and on the other hand if the disease can be recognized; early treatment for limb ischemia to prevent further complications. For both the patient and the national health care system, PCPs should take a leading role to evaluate and improve the main strategies to lower the risks and the health care costs, for both PAD and DM. The US national health care expenditures for cardiovascular disease meaning coronary heart disease, stroke, and PAD account for a large and increasing fraction of total US health care costs. Researches demonstrate that the costs for inpatient and outpatient PAD treatments are high, averaging $1868 per patient. Surgical inpatient treatment is accounted for the majority of the costs, averaging $1104 per PAD patient. To put these numbers into perspective, the $3.9 billion estimate for total Medicare paid PAD-related care is comparable with the estimates of Medicare expenditures for cardiac dysrhythmias ($2.7 billion), congestive heart failure ($ 3.9 billion), and cerebrovascular disease ($3.7 billion) [17]. Earlier recognition of PAD by patients and clinicians is an opportunity to reduce costs via initiation of preventive care strategies. Since PAD is a chronic medical condition, a comprehensive care plan should be made for patients with PAD, and this plan should include periodic clinical evaluation by a primary care physician with an awareness of vascular disease care. In addition, despite the current availability of guideline-based preventive therapy, its use is not optimal, and adverse vascular events and associated hospitalizations remain high among PAD patients. Studies suggest that the per-patient costs for PAD treatment are more than necessary compared to other cardiovascular disease presentations. At this point, awareness of both patients and physicians is of great importance. Continuing care focuses on reducing cardiovascular risk with medical therapy, optimizing functional status with structured exercise, and then revascularization when indicated. The further care plan is customized to the needs of the patient. In this context, it is reported that the economic burden of the disease can be reduced by intervening the preventable complications. Besides medical treatment with antiplatelet agents, control of hypertension, hyperglycemia and dyslipidemia, smoking cessation and structured exercise appear to be interventions with moderate / high levels of evidence. In addition to these direct costs, coronary heart disease (CHD) and PAD can lead to productivity costs associated with significant morbidity and mortality.

National Health and Wellness Surveys in the EU and USA reported significant workplace deterioration in patients with PAD based on absenteeism, availability, overall loss of work productivity, and activity impairment [18].

CHD and PAD represent a significant medical and economic burden worldwide. Although some progress has been reported to improve survival, morbidity, quality of life and direct costs of thrombotic disease, it is high and increasing. Results may be improved by using more antithrombotics and medication / lifestyle changes recommended by the guidelines to control modifiable cardiovascular risk factors. Earlier use of preventive care (e.g., atherosclerosis risk reduction), outpatient claudication treatments (e.g., supervised exercise), and durable revascularization interventions by being referred on time should be evaluated as strategies to both improve health and limit national health care costs [19, 20].

AWARENESS

In primary health care centers, the physicians must keep in mind that one in every two person is unaware of their diabetes condition, which can be classified as a silent killer; since unawareness and ignorance leads to mortal complications. Almost half of people with DM are not diagnosed (and treated) for an indefinite period and may develop complications during this time. For this reason, guidelines often recommend screening for DM in people over 40 to 45 years of age and / or with high risk factors such as a family history of diabetes, overweight (obesity), abdominal obesity (increased waist circumference) and hypertension. Managing DM is complex, time consuming and continuous. For this reason, PCPs face difficulties in meeting the changing medical needs of those with the disease. With limited access to the most up-to-date tools and treatments, the challenge becomes even more daunting when there are support staff, especially diabetes educators. There are currently available guidelines based on their extensive use to provide PCPs and their teams with clinical practice recommendations to facilitate decision-making in their daily real-world practice. The guidelines contain recommendations for the prevention of DM, along with some specific guidelines on this topic. Overall, all agree that a structured prevention program is needed for people with moderate hyperglycemia "prediabetes" [22-23].

Screening means a call to action: This process is very valuable to identify people with undiagnosed DM who would benefit from early treatment, as well as people with moderate hyperglycemia "prediabetes" who would benefit from a diabetes prevention program. Those diagnosed with diabetes should still be managed according to the guideline [21-23].

From this point of view in primary care, the first step is medical history taking which has a great importance in the first encounter. The family history of diabetes is an important clue. The second is the review of previous wounds, vascular treatments or evaluations, ulcerations and asking about pain especially while walking. Diagnostic criteria recommended by WHO (World Health Organization) and IDF (International Diabetes Federation) should be used in primary care. In particular, HbA1c should be considered as a diagnostic test. A standard HbA1c test should be performed in every primary care clinic, as it will also be necessary to decide on the treatment and monitor the disease and the effectiveness of the treatment. In addition, the guidelines recognize diabetes education as one of the cornerstones of diabetic patient management. The diabetic and PAD complications are more commonly represented as the incidence rises. Among diabetic patients 15-25% face vascular problems, one of which is foot ulcers ending 80% with non-traumatic lower-extremity amputation (LEA) [24]. We have to keep in mind that the progression of PAD is faster in diabetic patients leading to functional limitation that ends with lower extremity revascularization and amputation so they must be followed up more frequently. Healthcare providers have a unique opportunity in primary care to reduce the disease burden in this population. Early diagnosis and treatment of PAD in patients with diabetes is critical to reduce the risk of cardiovascular events, minimize the risk of long-term disability, and improve quality of life. Diagnosis of PAD in diabetic patients necessitates a versatile treatment approach that includes aggressive risk factor modification, antiplatelet therapy and revascularization procedures [6].

Amputation effects the quality of life for both patients and caregivers and is likely to lead to other amputations. The diabetic patients in the absence of symptoms may have worse prognosis for late complications when compared to the non-diabetics. The physician should not exclude PAD even if the patient does not have symptoms; they may have asymptomatic neuropathy, peripheral artery disease, pre-ulcerative signs or even an ulcer that is not recognized. Visual inspection can give clinician clues; such as, signs of vascular pathologies like dependent rubor (the patient sitting and legs hanging down), the loss of hair on the legs, pallor of the foot on elevated position, dry skin usually cool and cracked, toenails dystrophic or fungal infections. Fissures and ulcerations can be seen in the interdigital areas also. Physical examinations including palpation of pedal pulses and the loss of protective sensation will address the diabetic polyneuropathy. If neuropathy is present, further examinations must be planned to reveal the causes. In such cases, patient education is of great importance in addition to the awareness and strict follow-up of the doctor. To ensure adequate self-care skills, it is important to assess whether the person with diabetes (or any close family member or caregiver) understands the messages and is motivated to take action and follow the advice. In addition, healthcare professionals providing these instructions should receive periodic training to improve their skills in caring for people at high risk of foot ulcers [24].

Education, delivered in a structured, organized and repetitive fashion, is thought to play an important role in the prevention of diabetic foot ulcers. The most important goal here is to develop a patient's foot self-care knowledge and self-protection behavior, and to develop motivation and skills to facilitate adherence to this behavior. For this reason, the justification for performing a foot examination on the entire surface of both feet, including the areas between the toes, should be explained to the patient. People with diabetes, especially those at high risk, should learn how to recognize foot ulcers and ulcerative symptoms and be aware of the steps to take when problems arise. The healthcare team, particularly family physicians, plays a major role in providing structured training individually or in small groups [25].

PAD patient assessment in primary care includes patient history, physical examination, and intermittent claudication questionnaire focusing on atherothrombotic diseases. By the patient's medical history and examination: Ischemic rest pain, impaired walking function, intermittent claudication, diminished lower extremity pulses, lower extremity gangrene, recurrent and non-healing lower extremity wounds, dependent rubor and pallor on the elevation position can be seen. The clinical importance of early diagnosis and treatment of lower extremity peripheral artery disease as a manifestation of generalized atherothrombotic disease has been increasingly recognized in recent years. The recommended testing for these groups of patients in AHA/ACC (American Heart Association/ American College of Cardiology) guidelines are; resting ABI measurement as a diagnostic test with Doppler Ultrasound which is non-invasive, inexpensive, reliable and practical for physicians in primary care centers. Lower extremity hemodynamics are assessed in this examination by measurement of the highest systolic pressure in both legs from the dorsalis pedis artery and posterior tibial recurrent arteries and both arms brachial pressures than calculating the ratio of the highest pressures. ABI is the most common method of testing stenosis, with a sensitivity as high as 95-97%. This is method is defined as an efficient method of objectively documenting the presence and severity of lower extremity PAD by determination of ABI, which can be done in a physician's office with inexpensive equipment. When compared to angiography, the sensitivity of the ABI is about 90%, and the specificity is about 98% for stenosis of 50% or more in leg arteries. Ankle-brachial index range between 1.0 to 1.3 are classified as normal, which means no blockage. 0.9 to 1.0 means there is borderline blockage and extra testing may be needed for exercise ankle-branchial index. Less than 0.9 is abnormal and accepted as a diagnosis of PAD, where additional testing with ultrasound or angiography should be planned. If the results are, <0.4 it is called as severe PAD and the arteries should be viewed with angiography and medical treatment or surgery may be needed.

The studies stated that the WHO IC (Intermittent Claudication) questionnaire could be only diagnostic for a portion of the patients with PAD when compared to the ABI measurement. This suggests that the questionnaire was used for a specific purpose to identify symptomatic PAD, but not screening for early PAD. It has been investigated that some patients with PAD may not be diagnosed when physicians only try to detect it with the IC questionnaire (and / or clinical examination, respectively). Detecting ABI is a bit more time consuming than using questionnaires and learning how to do it is necessary, but it is also a viable and effective screening method in a population. Thus, determining a low ABI values is a useful tool to identify PAD in the hands of not only specialists but also general practitioners. It will be an important part of an effective strategy for PAD diagnose in primary care [26]. In order to have successful results, for good management of the patient in primary care close follow-up and blood sugar regulation has to be established regardless of the method used for treatment.

ASSOCIATED CONDITIONS AND COMORBIDITIES

The life style, daily routines, smoking, nutrition behaviors, exercise habits, general body condition, familial predispositions, psychologic disorders, physiologic and biologic markers, other existing illnesses or pre-illnesses like prediabetes are gateways for the practitioner to plan monitoring every other patient individually. Smoking cessation and early intervention for hypertension and hyperglycemia are found to be the most important ones not only for PAD but also for Cerebral Vascular Diseases.

The key point here is to keep in mind that coexisting diabetes in patients with PAD makes the situation much more complicated for the patient, caregiver and the health professionals with increased risk of cardiovascular and cerebrovascular events, which poses a major public health problem, and a challenge. The coexistence of DM and PAD requires much more attention and is important. Since PAD can be asymptomatic until it progresses, attention should be paid to comorbidities and necessary interventions should be performed in high risk patients group. It occurs at an earlier age and progresses more rapidly in those with non-diabetic patients. It is usually more severe and revascularization procedure may not be recommended to all patients, often when necessary. Moreover, the outcome after revascularization procedures is worse and many patients progress towards a major amputation [27].

It is well known that poor glycemic control is a predisposition for infections and poor wound healing associated with micro and macro angiopathy. According to clinical and experimental evidence, diabetic ulcers do not make regular and reliable progress in wound healing. As is known, complications such as infection, thrombosis and ischemia may occur even during normal wound healing process. In the case of diabetic ulcers, the healing impairment is caused by several internal factors (neuropathy, vascular problems complicating other diabetes-related systemic effects) and external factors (wound infection, callus formation and excessive pressure to the area). Traditionally, this group of predisposing abnormalities in diabetes has been referred to as the pathogenic triad of neuropathy, ischemia, and trauma. However, it is not so simple, one pathogenic abnormality can lead to another and vicious pathogenicity cycles can occur in the diabetic foot. Based on clinical and experimental evidence, there is no regular and reliable improvement in wound healing of diabetic ulcers. Although there are care guidelines determined by various international working groups, it is observed that professionals generally do not comply with these guidelines and the choice of patient approach and management is still influenced by individual characteristics and opinions [26].

Although thought to be related, the link between glucose control and the development or stabilization of neuropathic abnormalities has not been conclusively proven. Checking glucose concentrations, treating infection and correcting perfusion abnormalities is as important as a comprehensive evaluation of the patient and the wound. Even after the wound is completely closed, constant attention is required in terms of glucose control, daily attention to any loss of skin integrity and tissue regeneration. Prevention of wound recurrence is also critical [28]. Diabetes a leading cause of non-traumatic major and minor amputations worldwide recognized as the lower extremity amputations (LEA) predictor, causing a wide health and financial burden. Given the large number of diabetics known and increasing predicted numbers, there is an urgent need to develop and implement coordinated and multisectoral strategies to combat diabetes and complications. It has been shown that DM and its co-occurring PAD can be prevented or delayed through lifestyle modification or the administration of certain pharmacological treatments. Although the effectiveness of prevention in quality of life, disease burden, morbidity and mortality is clear in DM and vascular complications, translating these findings targeting high-risk individuals into national policies remains a challenge. The attempts made so far aim at unhealthy diet and physical inactivity as the drivers of overweight and obesity, the most important modifiable risk factors. In addition, it should not be forgotten that fighting with smoking for PAD [29]. Patients with diabetes have a varied, yet overall increased risk of LEA with an incidence of 50-500 per 100,000. Peripheral neuropathy and vascular diseases are main reasons for diabetic foot ulcers (DFU) subsequently leading to a higher rate of LEA which can lead to mortality up to 22% in diabetic patients. This is often attributed to the relatively advanced age and high prevalence of cardiovascular comorbidities in amputation as a sign of end-stage disease and multi-organ failure; but it has also been demonstrated as a lack of maintenance [26, 29].

It is known that the duration and severity of diabetes are associated with the incidence and extent of PAD. The degree of diabetic control is an important risk factor for PAD; with each 1% increase in glycosylated hemoglobin, the risk of PAD increased by 28%. There is a positive trend between PAD severity and amputation rate in patients with diabetes. Therefore, successful glycemic control and a careful medical intervention program in patients can prevent most limb amputations [30]. The amputations, both minor and major, effects the patient's quality of life and have higher risk for re-amputation and mortality in the long-term. The patient's immunosuppression and impaired blood flow to DFU make conservative treatment with antibiotics difficult and usually mandate extensive, repeated debridement or eventual amputation. In addition to systematic reviews and meta-analyzes supporting these findings, outcomes in diabetes mellitus often depend on patient compliance, influenced by their socio-economic or cultural background, and further studies are needed in these groups [31].

Glycemic control alone is not always enough for management strategy, also lowering blood pressure using medications, lipid-lowering with nutrition strategies and medications, antiplatelet therapy, exercise conditioning, and ensuring continued smoking cessation are vital for reducing the progression of diabetic complications or delaying the progression as similar for PAD. Because although studies have shown that strict glycemic control reduces the risk of developing microvascular diseases including retinopathy and neuropathy in diabetic patients, it has not been shown to reduce the risk of macrovascular complications. In patients with diabetes and PAD, blood glucose levels should be controlled aggressively with a hemoglobin A1c target of 7.0%, or as close to 6% as possible (level of evidence C). In addition, the effect of strict glucose control on cardiovascular outcomes in patients with PAD is not fully known. Although some studies have not shown a risk reduction for PAD with strict glycemic control, the effects of providing glycemic control are clear in maintaining low coronary and cerebrovascular events. Therefore, the focus of treatment in these patients should be aggressive and appropriate management of other cardiovascular risk factors such as hyperlipidemia, hypertension, smoking, including antiplatelet therapy, in order to reduce macrovascular complications [5, 32, 33].

Another point is the psychological status of the patient. Diabetic people show higher rate of depressive symptoms and anxiety. Depressive symptoms are more often when the disease progresses and complications occur. It becomes harder for the patients having appropriate cooperation with the health professionals caused by their additional psychological problems or psychiatric diseases. Patients' self-care will be low with depression. In addition, smoking cessation, adaption to nutritional advices and exercise programs will not be gracious for these individuals. Studies also reveal a correlation between PAD and Major Depressive Disorder. Peripheral artery disease and major depression often coexist among people who are demographically at risk for atherosclerotic disease. These findings highlight that depression is a potential mediator of proatherosclerotic events in this potentially at-risk patient population, and a greater focus is needed on concomitant mental health diagnoses among patients with known PAD.

Although physical exercise is generally encouraged in patients with intermittent claudication, it is known that compliance is low. Difficulty in performing the exercise may be related to the psychological characteristics of patients with limping. Symptoms of anxiety and depression are common in peripheral arterial patients. Depression symptoms in PAD are associated with personal barriers to exercise, while anxiety symptoms are not. Among patients with IC, the main barriers to physical activity are exercise-related pain and other illnesses [34-36].

There are several studies about smoking associated with increased risk of Type 2 diabetes. A number of studies have evaluated the relationship between smoking and the prevalence of glucose abnormalities, suggesting that active smoking may independently be associated with glucose intolerance, impaired fasting glucose, and Type 2 diabetes; therefore, smoking may be a modifiable risk factor for Type 2 diabetes. Some studies reveal consistent evidence of the increased incidence of diabetes associated with active smoking. However, studies that include detailed measurements and corrections of potential confounding factors such as socioeconomic status, education and exercise are needed to investigate whether the relationship with smoking is causal [37]. Nicotine causes insensitivity to insulin with the other chemicals in cigarette. In addition, nicotine patches have been found to decrease the effect of insulin. Smoking severely aggravates glucose tolerance and the insulin sensitivity index. It has been shown in studies that smoking is one of the most important risk factors for PAD. And also it has been found that smoking increases the risk of PAD several times and is a higher-impact risk factor for PAD than coronary artery disease [38].

Studies have shown that circulating microRNAs are irregular in smokers and are associated with the presence of PAD. In a study investigating wound healing, active smoking was associated with higher rates of incomplete wound healing in patients with critical limb ischemia undergoing endovascular interventions. Due to that, smoking cessation, a cause for both diabetes and PAD, should be an emergent action for the physician as a primary prevention strategy [38-42].

Sedentary life style and obesity are strongly correlated with diabetes hypertension and PAD. Approximately, 90% of diabetic patients are overweight (BMI > 25 kg/m^2). Weight loss can have an important impact in prevention for diabetes and correlated illnesses like hypertension, PAD and many others. Therefore, even just a moderate weight loss can have an immense impact in controlling diabetes as well as many complications. Achieving moderate weight loss combined with increased activity may improve insulin sensitivity and glycemic control in patients with type 2 diabetes and prevent the development of type 2 diabetes in high-risk individuals (i.e., those with impaired glucose tolerance). In addition, even mild weight reduction has been shown to be beneficial in improving insulin resistance, dyslipidemia and hypertension control. Obesity is associated with increased relative risks for overall mortality and cardiovascular disease. Weight control is also recommended to form a key feature of the overall management strategy in PAD. It has also been shown that body mass index is directly related to total cholesterol, blood pressure, and blood sugar levels. Abdominal fat distribution is associated with total body obesity, and this should be considered in peripheral arterial occlusive disease regardless of concomitant cardiovascular risk factors. Weight loss can increase insulin sensitivity and increase HDL-Cholesterol. Losing weight can also increase walking distance, as it will reduce the limitation of movement. An optimal diet plan and weight loss goal should be given to every overweight PAD patient [43-45].

Strict life style modifications again comes as an essential and emerging act. Lifestyle modification is the most appropriate intervention for the prevention of PAD complications and sequelae. Among these, nutrition and exercise are in the first place. Various risk factors have been identified in the pathophysiology of peripheral artery disease and need to be modified to reduce them. Smoking, hyperlipidemia, hypertension, and diabetes are among the proven risk factors for the development of peripheral artery disease, so it has been shown to be effective in preventing smoking cessation, lipid control, blood pressure control and associated morbidity [46]. Nutritional behaviors should be examined, as healthy diet is necessary for weight goals, glycemic targets, blood pressure, lipid targets that delay or prevent from diabetic complications and microvascular diseases. Dietary modification in PAD patients should be the first intervention to control abnormal lipid levels [Level of evidence B]. In symptomatic PAD patients, statins should be the primary agents for lowering LDL cholesterol levels to reduce the risk of cardiovascular events [Evidence Level A]. It is stated that patients with any atherosclerotic disease should be on a low-fat diet, animal products with high fat content and dairy products should be avoided. There is also evidence of the benefit of a 'Mediterranean' type diet rich in fruits, nuts, vegetables, fish and monounsaturated vegetable oils. Dietary changes should be made according to the patient's needs and comorbidities. Consulting a dietician can often be helpful, especially for patients with significant comorbidities. According to guidelines, patients should follow a diet low in carbohydrate and fat. Saturated fat intake should be limited to less than 7% of total calorie intake, and trans fats should be reduced. Nutrition with whole grains should be recommended with a fiber intake of 14 g / 1000 kcal in the daily diet. Lipid-lowering guidelines of the National Education Cholesterol Program recommend that patients with PAD should have an LDL cholesterol level of 100 mg / dL and be given treatment for high serum triglyceride levels [47-49]. A possible inverse association between better adherence to the Mediterranean diet and the risk of symptomatic

PAD has been reported in the randomized clinical trial. A Mediterranean-style diet may be effective in primary and secondary prevention of PAD, but further experimental studies are required to clarify this relationship. Similar results were found with the consumption of fruits and vegetables [50, 51].

The exercise training is vital as it improves walking ability and physical functions, vitality and general health with positive effects on mental health. The effects on reducing the risk of LEI (Lower extremity ischemia), CVD, or mortality could not be proven yet, but maximal and pain-free walking distance, thus quality of life is improved significantly; also, there has been less need for caregivers. There is evidence from studies that exercise programs provide significant benefits over placebo or usual care in improving both pain-free walking and maximum walking distance in people with leg pain from IC. Although exercise does not improve ABI and there is no evidence yet of the effect of exercise on amputation or mortality, it is recognized that exercise can improve quality of life compared to placebo or usual care. According to the results of the studies, it is recommended that patients with PAD exercise three times a week at a level that causes a moderate limp and then rest. Exercise regimens such as treadmill walking are said to be sufficient. Supervised exercise regimens have been found to give better results and are appropriate to recommend to patients, but a minimum of 3 months of exercise is required to reap the benefits of exercise. In patients with PAD, a structured community or home-based exercise program with behavioral modification techniques can be beneficial to improve walking ability and functional status. On the verge of these results, clinical practice guidelines advise the recommendation of structured home walking programs with weekly group-mediated cognitive behavioral intervention for PAD patients who do not have access to supervised exercise [52-59].

Patient educations' importance cannot be ignored for most of the chronic illnesses. Self-care in diabetes and PAD must be defined as an evolutionary process for development of knowledge and awareness by learning to survive with the complex nature of the diabetes. As the patient or caregivers majorly handle daily care, the needs of the patients should be managed in their social context and this must be a guide to the patient educations content [60]. By this way, the patients and their caregivers learning skills improve to better management of their diabetes while their daily routines continue with daily changes and needs. These needs differ for each individual, which are in fact determined by many factors like; daily routines, employment, family life, education and the community they are living in. This also improves the decision-making thus improving their confidence and coping skills. The individuals' feeling of wellbeing lowers the anxiety while increasing the quality-of-life at the same time. On the contrary, if the patient's self-management and coping skills are not enough, psychiatric disorders like anxiety and depression will be inevitable [61].

Nutritional behaviors, physical activities and exercise training, blood sugar monitoring and applying medications, risk reduction, problem solving abilities and need for seeking medical care are the major points for patient education. Diabetes self-care gives the patients a real role in many dietary and lifestyle modifications with the support of healthcare professionals, and gives them self-confidence and a better behavior change. There is evidence from the researches that the participation of diabetic patients in diabetes self-management education shows a statistically significant decrease in A1C levels [62-64].

Also in PAD, it is known that managing the risk factors can reduce the risk of further cardiovascular damage. Therefore, the patients can do their best if they are aware of themselves. What can be done will be similar to those mentioned above for diabetes. Studies show that people with peripheral artery disease do not understand the causes of the disease, lack of belief that lifestyle interventions will have a positive effect on disease outcomes, and unrealistic expectations about the outcome of surgical interventions. Although the goals of PAD therapy depend on the severity of the disease, reducing the risk of cardiovascular morbidity and mortality is a primary concern for all patients with PAD, symptomatic or not. Improving functional status is an additional goal for patients with IC. Especially for patients with critical limb ischemia, preventing leg amputation, restoring mobility and reducing mortality are of great importance [65].

Managing patients with multiple conditions can be complex, especially when recommendations applicable to coexisting illnesses are discordant or interacting [66]. The guidelines are intended to define practices meeting the needs of patients in most, but not all, circumstances. The recommendations should not replace clinical judgment. That is the point why primary care and family physicians are important for not only screening and follow up but also for appropriate diagnosis and effective treatment of these patients.

IMPORTANCE OF PRIMARY HEALTHCARE

The primary healthcare professionals can ask why they should care about PAD? As we mentioned the primary care keeps a key role in the prevention of limb loss since they are the first point of contact for recognition, diagnosis and referral. Like many other illnesses, Diabetes is strongly associated with PAD. The major cause of death and complications in patients with type 2 diabetes is vascular. Approximately 60% of diabetics die due to cardiovascular disease, and have more severe complications like PAD and amputations. The combined prevalence of vascular disease, hypertension, and dyslipidemia are all serious burdens for a patient, as well as their families and even the worldwide health care system [67].

Silence of the symptoms can sometimes be the cause of the morbidity and mortality so the physicians should keep this in mind and plan the screening accordingly, making sure to address the particular needs of the patients. Lifestyle changes, control of blood pressure, blood sugar and lipids, and antiplatelet therapy are the main interventions, which can prevent, reduce the progression of type 2 diabetes, PAD, CVD and associated complications [68].

Through studies have unfortunately shown that, the use of secondary prevention and lifestyle counseling in patients with PAD has not become a usual practice yet as well as public awareness. Future researches must aim to improve the quality of life by secondary prevention and life style counseling for PAD patients before invasive treatments are needed. Healthcare with high quality provided by a large group of health care professionals supported by governments can provide PAD patients higher quality of life [69]. In addition to improving survival, a key goal of PAD management is to improve symptoms, functioning and quality of life which can only be assessed by the primary care physician's perspective; taking into account biological, psychological, and social aspects of their patients [70, 71].

Primary care physicians are in the best position to deliver this highly effective and evidence-based care, PAD awareness and the use of guidelines are essential to make use of this opportunity to benefit.

REFERENCES

[1]   Saeedi, P., Petersohn, I., Salpea, P., Malanda, B., Karuranga, S., Unwin, N., Colagiuri, S., Guariguata, L., Motala, A. A., Ogurtsova, K., Shaw, J. E., Bright, D., Williams, R., & IDF Diabetes Atlas Committee (2019). Global and regional diabetes prevalence estimates for 2019 and projections for 2030 and 2045: Results from the International Diabetes Federation Diabetes Atlas, 9th edition. *Diabetes research and clinical practice*, *157*, 107843. https://doi.org/10.1016/j.diabres.2019.107843.

[2]   Advocacy guide to the *IDF Diabetes Atlas* Ninth edition 2019. https://diabetesatlas.org/upload/resources/material/20191217_165723_2019_IDF_Advocacy_guide.pdf.

[3]   Parvar, S. L., Fitridge, R., Dawson, J., & Nicholls, S. J. (2018). Medical and lifestyle management of peripheral arterial disease. *Journal of vascular surgery*, 68(5), 1595–1606. https://doi.org/10.1016/j.jvs.2018.07.027.

[4]   Kügler, C. F., & Rudofsky, G. (2003). The challenges of treating peripheral arterial disease. *Vascular medicine* (London, England), 8(2), 109–114. https://doi.org/10.1191/1358863x03vm478ra.

[5]   Althouse, A. D., Abbott, J. D., Forker, A. D., Bertolet, M., Barinas-Mitchell, E., Thurston, R. C., Mulukutla, S., Aboyans, V., Brooks, M. M., & BARI 2D Study Group (2014). Risk factors for incident peripheral arterial disease in type 2 diabetes: results from the Bypass Angioplasty Revascularization Investigation in type 2 Diabetes (BARI 2D) Trial. *Diabetes care, 37*(5), 1346–1352. https://doi.org/ 10.2337/dc13-2303.

[6]   Firnhaber, J. M., & Powell, C. S. (2019). Lower Extremity Peripheral Artery Disease: Diagnosis and Treatment. *American family physician, 99*(6), 362–369.

[7]   Jude, E. B., Oyibo, S. O., Chalmers, N., & Boulton, A. J. (2001). Peripheral arterial disease in diabetic and nondiabetic patients: a comparison of severity and outcome. *Diabetes care, 24*(8), 1433–1437. https://doi.org/10.2337/diacare.24.8.1433.

[8]   Fowkes, F. G., Rudan, D., Rudan, I., Aboyans, V., Denenberg, J. O., McDermott, M. M., Norman, P. E., Sampson, U. K., Williams, L. J., Mensah, G. A., & Criqui, M. H. (2013). Comparison of global estimates of prevalence and risk factors for peripheral artery disease in 2000 and 2010: a systematic review and analysis. *Lancet (London, England), 382*(9901), 1329–1340. https://doi.org/10.1016/S0140-6736(13)61249-0.

[9]   Wattanakit, K., Folsom, A. R., Selvin, E., Weatherley, B. D., Pankow, J. S., Brancati, F. L., & Hirsch, A. T. (2005). Risk factors for peripheral arterial disease incidence in persons with diabetes: the Atherosclerosis Risk in Communities (ARIC) Study. *Atherosclerosis, 180*(2), 389–397. https://doi.org/10.1016/j.atherosclerosis. 2004.11. 024.

[10]   Marso, S. P., & Hiatt, W. R. (2006). Peripheral arterial disease in patients with diabetes. *Journal of the American College of Cardiology, 47*(5), 921–929. https://doi.org/10.1016/j.jacc.2005. 09.065.

[11]   Beckman, J. A., Paneni, F., Cosentino, F., & Creager, M. A. (2013). Diabetes and vascular disease: pathophysiology, clinical

consequences, and medical therapy: part II. *European heart journal*, *34*(31), 2444–2452. https://doi.org/10.1093/eurheartj/eht142.

[12] Aquino, R., Johnnides, C., Makaroun, M., Whittle, J. C., Muluk, V. S., Kelley, M. E., & Muluk, S. C. (2001). Natural history of claudication: long-term serial follow-up study of 1244 claudicants. *Journal of vascular surgery*, *34*(6), 962–970. https://doi.org/10.1067/mva.2001.119749.

[13] *American Diabetes Association Diagnosing Diabetes and Learning about Prediabetes*. [(accessed on 3 March 2020)]; Available online: http://www.diabetes.org/diabetes-basics/diagnosis/.

[14] Tuso P. (2014). Prediabetes and lifestyle modification: time to prevent a preventable disease. *The Permanente journal*, *18*(3), 88–93. https://doi.org/10.7812/TPP/14-002.

[15] Warren, B., Pankow, J. S., Matsushita, K., Punjabi, N. M., Daya, N. R., Grams, M., Woodward, M., & Selvin, E. (2017). Comparative prognostic performance of definitions of prediabetes: a prospective cohort analysis of the Atherosclerosis Risk in Communities (ARIC) study. *The lancet. Diabetes & endocrinology*, *5*(1), 34–42. https://doi.org/10.1016/S2213-8587(16)30321-7.

[16] Emerging Risk Factors Collaboration, Sarwar, N., Gao, P., Seshasai, S. R., Gobin, R., Kaptoge, S., Di Angelantonio, E., Ingelsson, E., Lawlor, D. A., Selvin, E., Stampfer, M., Stehouwer, C. D., Lewington, S., Pennells, L., Thompson, A., Sattar, N., White, I. R., Ray, K. K., & Danesh, J. (2010). Diabetes mellitus, fasting blood glucose concentration, and risk of vascular disease: a collaborative meta-analysis of 102 prospective studies. *Lancet (London, England)*, *375*(9733), 2215–2222. https://doi.org/10.1016/S0140-6736(10)60484-9.

[17] *Medicare and Medicaid Statistical Supplement*, 2004, Table 28.

[18] Marrett, E., DiBonaventura, M. d., & Zhang, Q. (2013). Burden of peripheral arterial disease in Europe and the United States: a patient survey. *Health and quality of life outcomes*, 11, 175. https://doi.org/10.1186/1477-7525-11-175.

[19] Hirsch, A. T., Hartman, L., Town, R. J., & Virnig, B. A. (2008). National health care costs of peripheral arterial disease in the Medicare population. *Vascular medicine (London, England)*, *13*(3), 209–215. https://doi.org/10.1177/1358863X08089277.

[20] Rupert Bauersachs, Uwe Zeymer, Jean-Baptiste Brière, Caroline Marre, Kevin Bowrin, Maria Huelsebeck, "Burden of Coronary Artery Disease and Peripheral Artery Disease: A Literature Review," *Cardiovascular Therapeutics*, vol. 2019, Article ID 8295054, 9 pages, 2019.

[21] International Diabetes Federation. *IDF Diabetes Atlas. 8th ed.* International Diabetes Federation; Brussels, Belgium: 2017. pp. 9–44. https://diabetesatlas.org/upload/resources/previous/files/8/IDF _ DA_8e-EN-final.pdf.

[22] International Diabetes Federation. *Recommendations for Managing Type 2 Diabetes in Primary Care,* 2017. www.idf.org/managing-type2-diabetes.

[23] Aschner P. (2017). New IDF clinical practice recommendations for managing type 2 diabetes in primary care. *Diabetes research and clinical practice*, 132, 169–170. https://doi.org/10.1016/j.diabres. 2017.09.002.

[24] Cascini, S., Agabiti, N., Davoli, M., Uccioli, L., Meloni, M., Giurato, L., Marino, C., & Bargagli, A. M. (2020). Survival and factors predicting mortality after major and minor lower-extremity amputations among patients with diabetes: a population-based study using health information systems. *BMJ open diabetes research & care*, 8(1), e001355. https://doi.org/10.1136/bmjdrc-2020-001355.

[25] Schaper, N. C., van Netten, J. J., Apelqvist, J., Bus, S. A., Hinchliffe, R. J., Lipsky, B. A., & IWGDF Editorial Board (2020). Practical Guidelines on the prevention and management of diabetic foot disease (IWGDF 2019 update). *Diabetes/metabolism research and reviews*, *36 Suppl 1*, e3266. https://doi.org/10.1002/dmrr.3266.

[26] Diehm, C., Schuster, A., Allenberg, J. R., Darius, H., Haberl, R., Lange, S., Pittrow, D., von Stritzky, B., Tepohl, G., & Trampisch, H. J. (2004). High prevalence of peripheral arterial disease and co-

morbidity in 6880 primary care patients: cross-sectional study. *Atherosclerosis*, *172*(1), 95–105. https://doi.org/10.1016/s0021-9150(03)00204-1.

[27] Guan, H., Liu, Z. M., Li, G. W., Guo, X. H., Xu, Z. R., Zou, D. J., Xing, H. L., Liu, W., Sheng, Z. Y., Tian, H. M., Zhu, D. L., Yu, D. M., Zhuang, W. T., Chen, L. L., & Weng, J. P. (2007). Analysis of peripheral arterial obstructive disease related factors among diabetic population aged > or = 50. *Zhonghua yi xue za zhi*, *87*(1), 23–27.

[28] Falanga V. (2005). Wound healing and its impairment in the diabetic foot. *Lancet (London, England)*, *366*(9498), 1736–1743. https://doi.org/10.1016/S0140-6736(05)67700-8.

[29] Saeedi, P., Petersohn, I., Salpea, P., Malanda, B., Karuranga, S., Unwin, N., Colagiuri, S., Guariguata, L., Motala, A. A., Ogurtsova, K., Shaw, J. E., Bright, D., Williams, R., & IDF Diabetes Atlas Committee (2019). Global and regional diabetes prevalence estimates for 2019 and projections for 2030 and 2045: Results from the International Diabetes Federation Diabetes Atlas, 9th edition. *Diabetes research and clinical practice*, *157*, 107843. https://doi.org/10.1016/j.diabres.2019.107843.

[30] van Netten, J. J., Fortington, L. V., Hinchliffe, R. J., & Hijmans, J. M. (2016). Early Post-operative Mortality after Major Lower Limb Amputation: A Systematic Review of Population and Regional Based Studies. *European journal of vascular and endovascular surgery: the official journal of the European Society for Vascular Surgery*, *51*(2), 248–257. https://doi.org/10.1016/j.ejvs.2015.10.001.

[31] Rathnayake, A., Saboo, A., Malabu, U. H., & Falhammar, H. (2020). Lower extremity amputations and long-term outcomes in diabetic foot ulcers: A systematic review. *World journal of diabetes*, *11*(9), 391–399. https://doi.org/10.4239/wjd.v11.i9.391.

[32] Gandhi, S., Weinberg, I., Margey, R., & Jaff, M. R. (2011). Comprehensive medical management of peripheral arterial disease. *Progress in cardiovascular diseases*, *54*(1), 2–13. https://doi.org/10.1016/j.pcad.2011.02.004.

[33] Dormandy, J. A., Charbonnel, B., Eckland, D. J., Erdmann, E., Massi-Benedetti, M., Moules, I. K., Skene, A. M., Tan, M. H., Lefèbvre, P. J., Murray, G. D., Standl, E., Wilcox, R. G., Wilhelmsen, L., Betteridge, J., Birkeland, K., Golay, A., Heine, R. J., Korányi, L., Laakso, M., Mokán, M., ... PROactive Investigators (2005). Secondary prevention of macrovascular events in patients with type 2 diabetes in the PROactive Study (PROspective pioglitAzone Clinical Trial In macroVascular Events): a randomised controlled trial. *Lancet* (London, England), 366(9493), 1279–1289. https://doi.org/10.1016/S0140-6736(05)67528-9.

[34] Collins, M. M., Corcoran, P., & Perry, I. J. (2009). Anxiety and depression symptoms in patients with diabetes. *Diabetic medicine: a journal of the British Diabetic Association, 26*(2), 153–161. https://doi.org/10.1111/j.1464-5491.2008.02648.x.

[35] Columbo, J. A., Stone, D. H., Goodney, P. P., Nolan, B. W., Stableford, J. A., Brooke, B. S., Powell, R. J., & Finn, C. T. (2016). The Prevalence and Regional Variation of Major Depressive Disorder among Patients with Peripheral Arterial Disease in the Medicare Population. *Vascular and endovascular surgery*, 50(4), 235–240. https://doi.org/10.1177/1538574416644529.

[36] Ragazzo, L., Puech-Leao, P., Wolosker, N., de Luccia, N., Saes, G., Ritti-Dias, R. M., Cucato, G. G., Ferreira Kamikava, D. Y., & Zerati, A. E. (2021). Symptoms of anxiety and depression and their relationship with barriers to physical activity in patients with intermittent claudication. *Clinics* (Sao Paulo, Brazil), 76, e1802. https://doi.org/10.6061/clinics/2021/e1802.

[37] Willi, C., Bodenmann, P., Ghali, W. A., Faris, P. D., & Cornuz, J. (2007). Active smoking and the risk of type 2 diabetes: a systematic review and meta-analysis. *JAMA, 298*(22), 2654–2664. https://doi.org/10.1001/jama.298.22.2654.

[38] Frati, A. C., Iniestra, F., & Ariza, C. R. (1996). Acute effect of cigarette smoking on glucose tolerance and other cardiovascular risk factors. *Diabetes care, 19*(2), 112–118. https://doi.org/10.2337/diacare.19.2.112.

[39] Lu, J. T., & Creager, M. A. (2004). The relationship of cigarette smoking to peripheral arterial disease. *Reviews in cardiovascular medicine, 5(4), 189–193.*

[40] Pereira-da-Silva, T., Napoleão, P., Costa, M. C., Gabriel, A. F., Selas, M., Silva, F., Enguita, F. J., Ferreira, R. C., & Carmo, M. M. (2021). Cigarette Smoking, miR-27b Downregulation, and Peripheral Artery Disease: Insights into the Mechanisms of Smoking Toxicity. *Journal of clinical medicine, 10(4), 890.* https://doi.org/10.3390/jcm 10040890.

[41] Sagris, M., Kokkinidis, D. G., Lempesis, I. G., Giannopoulos, S., Rallidis, L., Mena-Hurtado, C., & Bakoyiannis, C. (2020). Nutrition, dietary habits, and weight management to prevent and treat patients with peripheral artery disease. *Reviews in cardiovascular medicine,* 21(4), 565–575. https://doi.org/10.31083/j.rcm.2020.04.202.

[42] Cheung, B. M., & Li, C. (2012). Diabetes and hypertension: is there a common metabolic pathway?. *Current atherosclerosis reports, 14*(2), 160–166. https://doi.org/10.1007/s11883-012-0227-2.

[43] Wild, S. H., & Byrne, C. D. (2006). ABC of obesity. Risk factors for diabetes and coronary heart disease. *BMJ (Clinical research ed.), 333*(7576), 1009–1011. https://doi.org/10.1136/bmj.39024.568738. 43.

[44] Gerhard-Herman MD, Gornik HL, Barrett C, Barshes NR, Corriere MA, Drachman DE, Fleisher LA, Fowkes FGR, Hamburg NM, Kinlay S, Lookstein R, Misra S, Mureebe L, Olin JW, Patel RAG, Regensteiner JG, Schanzer A, Shishehbor MH, Stewart KJ, Treat-Jacobson D, Walsh ME. 2016 AHA/ACC Guideline on the Management of Patients with Lower Extremity Peripheral Artery Disease: Executive Summary: A Report of the American College of Cardiology/American Heart Association Task Force on Clinical Practice Guidelines. *J Am Coll Cardiol.* 2017 Mar 21;69(11):1465-1508. doi: 10.1016/j.jacc.2016.11.008. Epub 2016 Nov 13. Erratum in: J Am Coll Cardiol. 2017 Mar 21;69(11):1520. PMID: 27851991.

[45] Klein, S., Sheard, N. F., Pi-Sunyer, X., Daly, A., Wylie-Rosett, J., Kulkarni, K., Clark, N. G., American Diabetes Association, North

American Association for the Study of Obesity, & American Society for Clinical Nutrition (2004). Weight management through lifestyle modification for the prevention and management of type 2 diabetes: rationale and strategies. A statement of the American Diabetes Association, the North American Association for the Study of Obesity, and the American Society for Clinical Nutrition. *The American journal of clinical nutrition*, 80(2), 257–263. https://doi.org/10.1093/ajcn/80.2.257.

[46] Aggarwal, S., Loomba, R. S., & Arora, R. (2012). Preventive aspects in peripheral artery disease. *Therapeutic advances in cardiovascular disease*, 6(2), 53–70. https://doi.org/10.1177/1753944712437359.

[47] Look AHEAD Research Group, Wing, R. R., Bolin, P., Brancati, F. L., Bray, G. A., Clark, J. M., Coday, M., Crow, R. S., Curtis, J. M., Egan, C. M., Espeland, M. A., Evans, M., Foreyt, J. P., Ghazarian, S., Gregg, E. W., Harrison, B., Hazuda, H. P., Hill, J. O., Horton, E. S., Hubbard, V. S., ... Yanovski, S. Z. (2013). Cardiovascular effects of intensive lifestyle intervention in type 2 diabetes. *The New England journal of medicine*, *369*(2), 145–154. https://doi.org/10.1056/NEJMoa1212914.

[48] Merchant, A. T., Hu, F. B., Spiegelman, D., Willett, W. C., Rimm, E. B., & Ascherio, A. (2003). Dietary fiber reduces peripheral arterial disease risk in men. *The Journal of nutrition*, 133(11), 3658–3663. https://doi.org/10.1093/jn/133.11.3658.

[49] American Diabetes Association (2010). Standards of medical care in diabetes--2010. *Diabetes care*, 33 Suppl 1(Suppl 1), S11–S61. https://doi.org/10.2337/dc10-S011.

[50] Ruiz-Canela, M., & Martínez-González, M. A. (2014). Lifestyle and dietary risk factors for peripheral artery disease. *Circulation journal: official journal of the Japanese Circulation Society*, 78(3), 553–559. https://doi.org/10.1253/circj.cj-14-0062.

[51] Heffron, S. P., Rockman, C. B., Adelman, M. A., Gianos, E., Guo, Y., Xu, J. F., & Berger, J. S. (2017). Greater Frequency of Fruit and Vegetable Consumption Is Associated With Lower Prevalence of Peripheral Artery Disease. *Arteriosclerosis, thrombosis, and vascular*

biology, 37(6), 1234–1240. https://doi.org/10.1161/ATVBAHA. 116.308474.

[52] Lane, R., Ellis, B., Watson, L., & Leng, G. C. (2014). Exercise for intermittent claudication. *The Cochrane database of systematic reviews*, (7), CD000990. https://doi.org/10.1002/14651858.CD0009 90.pub3.

[53] Nativel, M., Potier, L., Alexandre, L., Baillet-Blanco, L., Ducasse, E., Velho, G., Marre, M., Roussel, R., Rigalleau, V., & Mohammedi, K. (2018). Lower extremity arterial disease in patients with diabetes: a contemporary narrative review. *Cardiovascular diabetology*, *17*(1), 138. https://doi.org/10.1186/s12933-018-0781-1.

[54] Lane, R., Harwood, A., Watson, L., & Leng, G. C. (2017). Exercise for intermittent claudication. *The Cochrane database of systematic reviews,* 12(12), CD000990. https://doi.org/10.1002/14651858. CD000990.pub4.

[55] Hamburg, N. M., & Balady, G. J. (2011). Exercise rehabilitation in peripheral artery disease: functional impact and mechanisms of benefits. *Circulation*, 123(1), 87–97. https://doi.org/10.1161/ CIRCULATIONAHA.109.881888.

[56] Gerhard-Herman MD, Gornik HL, Barrett C, Barshes NR, Corriere MA, Drachman DE, Fleisher LA, Fowkes FGR, Hamburg NM, Kinlay S, Lookstein R, Misra S, Mureebe L, Olin JW, Patel RAG, Regensteiner JG, Schanzer A, Shishehbor MH, Stewart KJ, Treat-Jacobson D, Walsh ME. 2016 AHA/ACC guideline on the management of patients with lower extremity peripheral artery disease: executive summary: a report of the American College of Cardiology/American Heart Association Task Force on Clinical Practice Guidelines. *Circulation*. 2017;135:e686–e725. DOI: 10.1161/CIR.0000000000000470.

[57] Hirsch, A. T., Criqui, M. H., Treat-Jacobson, D., Regensteiner, J. G., Creager, M. A., Olin, J. W., Krook, S. H., Hunninghake, D. B., Comerota, A. J., Walsh, M. E., McDermott, M. M., & Hiatt, W. R. (2001). Peripheral arterial disease detection, awareness, and treatment in primary care. *JAMA*, 286(11), 1317–1324. https://doi.org/10.1001/jama.286.11.1317.

[58] McDermott M. M. (2018). Exercise Rehabilitation for Peripheral Artery Disease: A REVIEW. *Journal of cardiopulmonary rehabilitation and prevention*, 38(2), 63–69. https://doi.org/10.1097/HCR.0000000000000343.

[59] Hageman, D., Fokkenrood, H. J., Gommans, L. N., van den Houten, M. M., & Teijink, J. A. (2018). Supervised exercise therapy versus home-based exercise therapy versus walking advice for intermittent claudication. *The Cochrane database of systematic reviews*, 4(4), CD005263. https://doi.org/10.1002/14651858.CD005263.pub4.

[60] Shrivastava, S. R., Shrivastava, P. S., & Ramasamy, J. (2013). Role of self-care in management of diabetes mellitus. *Journal of diabetes and metabolic disorders*, *12*(1), 14. https://doi.org/10.1186/2251-6581-12-14.

[61] Simson, U., Nawarotzky, U., Friese, G., Porck, W., Schottenfeld-Naor, Y., Hahn, S., Scherbaum, W. A., & Kruse, J. (2008). Psychotherapy intervention to reduce depressive symptoms in patients with diabetic foot syndrome. *Diabetic medicine: a journal of the British Diabetic Association*, *25*(2), 206–212. https://doi.org/10.1111/j.1464-5491.2007.02370.x.

[62] AADE (2008). *AADE7 Self-Care Behaviors. The Diabetes educator*, 34(3), 445–449. https://doi.org/10.1177/0145721708316625.

[63] Chrvala, C. A., Sherr, D., & Lipman, R. D. (2016). Diabetes self-management education for adults with type 2 diabetes mellitus: A systematic review of the effect on glycemic control. *Patient education and counseling*, 99(6), 926–943. https://doi.org/10.1016/j.pec.2015.11.003.

[64] Powers, M. A., Bardsley, J., Cypress, M., Duker, P., Funnell, M. M., Hess Fischl, A., Maryniuk, M. D., Siminerio, L., & Vivian, E.

(2015). Diabetes Self-management Education and Support in Type 2 Diabetes: A Joint Position Statement of the American Diabetes Association, the American Association of Diabetes Educators, and the Academy of Nutrition and Dietetics. *Diabetes care*, 38(7), 1372–1382. https://doi.org/10.2337/dc15-0730.

[65] Khan, S., Cleanthis, M., Smout, J., Flather, M., & Stansby, G. (2005). Life-style modification in peripheral arterial disease. *European journal of vascular and endovascular surgery: the official journal of the European Society for Vascular Surgery*, 29(1), 2–9. https://doi.org/10.1016/j.ejvs.2004.09.020.

[66] Arnett, D. K., Goodman, R. A., Halperin, J. L., Anderson, J. L., Parekh, A. K., & Zoghbi, W. A. (2014). AHA/ACC/HHS strategies to enhance application of clinical practice guidelines in patients with cardiovascular disease and comorbid conditions: from the American Heart Association, American College of Cardiology, and US Department of Health and Human Services. *Circulation*, 130(18), 1662–1667. https://doi.org/10.1161/CIR.0000000000000128.

[67] Fox, C. S., Coady, S., Sorlie, P. D., D'Agostino, R. B., Sr, Pencina, M. J., Vasan, R. S., Meigs, J. B., Levy, D., & Savage, P. J. (2007). Increasing cardiovascular disease burden due to diabetes mellitus: the Framingham Heart Study. *Circulation*, 115(12), 1544–1550. https://doi.org/10.1161/CIRCULATIONAHA.106.658948.

[68] Gaede, P., Lund-Andersen, H., Parving, H. H., & Pedersen, O. (2008). Effect of a multifactorial intervention on mortality in type 2 diabetes. *The New England journal of medicine*, 358(6), 580–591. https://doi.org/10.1056/NEJMoa0706245

[69] Berger, J. S., & Ladapo, J. A. (2017). Underuse of Prevention and Lifestyle Counseling in Patients with Peripheral Artery Disease. *Journal of the American College of Cardiology*, 69(18), 2293–2300. https://doi.org/10.1016/j.jacc.2017.02.064

[70] Patel, K. K., Alturkmani, H., Gosch, K., Mena-Hurtado, C., Shishehbor, M. H., Peri-Okonny, P. A., Creager, M. A., Spertus, J. A., & Smolderen, K. G. (2020). Association of Diabetes Mellitus with Health Status Outcomes in Patients with Peripheral Artery

Disease: Insights from the PORTRAIT Registry. *Journal of the American Heart Association*, 9(22), e017103. https://doi.org/10.1161/JAHA.120.017103

[71] Burns, P., Gough, S., & Bradbury, A. W. (2003). Management of peripheral arterial disease in primary care. *BMJ (Clinical research ed.)*, 326(7389), 584–588. https://doi.org/10.1136/bmj.326.7389.584.

In: Peripheral Artery Disease ISBN: 978-1-53619-968-0
Editor: Jeremy D. Parks © 2021 Nova Science Publishers, Inc.

Chapter 3

RISK MANAGEMENT OF PERIPHERAL ARTERY DISEASE AT PRIMARY CARE SETTING

Gizem Limnili, MD and Nilgün Özçakar, MD*

Department of Family Medicine, Faculty of Medicine,
Dokuz Eylul University, İzmir, Turkey

ABSTRACT

Peripheral arterial disease (PAD) is a multifactorial process defined as a partial or complete occlusion of an artery in the upper or lower extremity due to atherosclerosis. It has similar risk factors to other cardiovascular diseases. The most important risk factors are diabetes mellitus, tobacco use, hypertension, and dyslipidemia. In addition, age, gender, ethnicity, inactivity and being overweight play a role. Since many people have asymptomatic PAD, known risk factors should be managed appropriately and in a timely manner. As a multifactorial disease, PAD requires multidimensional screening as well as easily applicable and accessible follow-up approaches. At this context, primary care physicians have an important position in screening undiagnosed asymptomatic PAD

* Corresponding Author's E-mail: gizem.limnili@deu.edu.tr.

and in monitoring patients with explained increased cardiovascular risk due to PAD.

Risk factors - Smoking increases risk of PAD up to a 10-fold. A systematic review suggests that half of all PADs are attributable to smoking. It was concluded that heavier smokers were more likely to develop PAD than light smokers, and that former smokers had a steadily increased risk compared to never smokers. Exposure to passive smoking has also been shown to promote changes leading to atherosclerosis. Diabetes has been shown to increase the risk of PAD 2-4 times. Poor diabetic control is associated with an increased risk of PAD. The risk of developing PAD is proportional to the severity and duration of diabetes. Dyslipidemia is correlated with accelerated PAD. Dyslipidemia management by diet, exercise, and/or medication is associated with a major reduction in cardiovascular diseases and stroke. Hypertension can increase risk of developing PAD. High blood pressure increases the risk of intermittent claudication, the most common symptom of PAD. Other risk factors can be listed as genetics leading to risk factors for PAD such as diabetes and hypertension but there have been no specific genes or gene mutations directly associated with them. The prevalence and outcome of peripheral artery disease shows differences with age and gender of the patients.

Considering all these risk factors in the population, family physicians have also a crucial role to arise PAD awareness among patients and general population. Increased awareness could enable earlier, appropriate and effective management of PAD and adherence to secondary prevention strategies for the modification of PAD risk factors at primary health care settings. This section will review PAD risk management and the role of family physician in primary care.

INTRODUCTION

Peripheral artery disease (PAD), which is due to atherosclerosis, is a multifactorial process defined as partial or complete occlusion of an artery in the upper or lower extremities. Its risk factors are similar to other cardiovascular diseases [1]. However, there are differences in the incidence and ranking of some risk factors [2]. Risk factors include age, gender, ethnicity, inactivity and being overweight, diabetes mellitus, tobacco use, hypertension and dyslipidemia. While factors such as poverty, industrialization, and infection could plausibly affect the development of PAH, aging of the population and an increase in traditional cardiovascular risk factors such as smoking, diabetes and hypertension will likely be the main cause [3].

The risk index and categories for 10-year mortality rates in patients with lower extremity peripheral artery disease are listed in Table 1 and Table 2.

Table 1. Risk index for 10-year mortality rates in patients with lower extremity peripheral artery disease

Risk factors	Points
Renal dysfunction	+ 12
Heart failure	+ 7
Age > 65 years	+ 5
Hypercholesterolemia	+ 5
ST-segment changes on ECG	+ 5
Ankle-brachial index < 0.6	+ 4
Q-waves on ECG	+ 4
Cerebrovascular disease	+ 3
Diabetes mellitus	+ 3
Pulmonary disease	+ 3
Statin use	− 6
Aspirin use	− 4
Beta blocker use	− 4

Table 2. Risk categories and associated 10-year mortality [5]

Risk category	Points	Associated 10-year mortality
Low	< 0	22.1%
Low-intermediate	0 to 5	32.2%
High-intermediate	6 to 9	45.8%
High	> 9	70.4%

AHA (2017) recommended screening the patients for PAD if they are in one of these groups:

- Age ≥70 years (no need for an additional risk factor)
- Age 50 to 69 years with a history of smoking or diabetes

- Age 40 to 49 with diabetes and at least one other risk factor for atherosclerosis
- Known atherosclerosis at other sites (e.g., coronary, carotid, renal artery disease) [4].

Age

The prevalence of PAD increases progressively from the age of 40 [6]. The relationship between PAD prevalence and age dramatically increases after the age of 70 [7]. Individuals over 70 are at a significantly increased risk for PAD due to age alone, while risk for those who are younger is due to other factors [8]. In addition, traditional risk factors for PAD may be absent in patients older than 80 years, particularly those with infrapopliteal disease [9]. As a result, PAD is a growing clinical problem due to an aging population worldwide. Although there is no additional risk factor for elderly patients, it is recommended to be screened for PAH; those with a history of smoking or diabetes and those at risk of atherosclerosis should be screened at an earlier age. [4.] Also in a metanalysis the prevalence of peripheral artery disease was relatively higher in low- and middle-income countries (LMICS) than in high income countries (HICS) in young people, but became lower from the age of 50 years, which might be related to a relatively lower life expectancy in LMICs than in HICs [10]. In primary care settings, the family physicians should be aware of age-related risk factors of the patients.

Gender

According to previous studies, like other cardiovascular diseases, PAD is more common in men. However, prevalence of PAD in women has not been completely evaluated. In population-based studies, the prevalence of PAD in women is at least as high as in men in all age groups, but increases significantly after the age of 70 compared to men of the same age [11, 12].

In some reviews focused on gender differences in different age groups, PAD risk was significantly more in women [13, 14]. According to a study of World Health Organization (WHO) regions, prevalence was higher in females, especially at younger ages in low-/middle-income regions [1]. Apart from the increased risk of PAD in women, there are different studies on the prevalence of PAD-related problems. For example, in a study, the prevalence of severe limb ischemia was 13.2 percent in females and 4.3 percent in males. The difference was likely related to hypercholesterolemia, metabolic syndrome, and diabetes mellitus which were found to be more common in the female patients [12]. On the other hand, there is a large review suggesting that the first occurrence of PAD is most often detected in men aged 50 to 59, with a two-fold increase compared to women [15]. It is unknown whether hormone replacement therapy has any effect on the development of PAD in postmenopausal women. Nevertheless, a study among women using hormone replacement therapy found that despite the increased prevalence of various atherosclerotic risk factors, they were significantly less likely to have PAD [16].

Ethnicity

The prevalence of PAD varies among ethnicities. The prevalence is higher in African Americans than non-Hispanic White Americans [17, 18]. The difference does not appear to be completely explained by differences in the prevalence of risk factors for atherosclerosis among different ethnicities [18]. African and Hispanic Americans have higher rates of diabetes and hypertension, whereas White Americans are more likely to have hypercholesterolemia [19]. In a multiethnic Asian (Chinese, Malays, and Indians) population study, PAD was present in 4.3 percent of the population [20]. A systematic review identified 14 studies comparing prevalence between South Asian and White European individuals and found a significantly lower risk of PAD in those from South Asian with coronary artery disease and diabetes [21]. In a systemic review, the

Western Pacific region (WPR) had the largest share of global peripheral artery disease cases (74.08 million, 95% CI 51.84–109.30), whereas the Eastern Mediterranean Region (EMR) had the least (14.67 million, 10.04–22.48). The prevalence of peripheral artery disease was highest in the European Region (7.99%, 5.10–13.41) and lowest in the African Region (4.06%, 2.90–5.91). More than two thirds of the global peripheral artery disease cases were concentrated in 15 individual countries, China, India, and the USA had the largest numbers of cases. The prevalence of peripheral artery disease was relatively higher in low- and middle-income countries (LMICs) than in high-income countries (HICs) in young people, but became lower from the age of 50 years, which might be related to a relatively lower life expectancy in LMICs than in HICs [10].

Family History and Genetic Factors

Atherosclerotic disease is likely the result of many genes interacting with each other and with the environment [22]. Families identified with early-onset atherosclerosis have an increased risk of PAD, but no single genetic markers for PAD have been identified in this population. Studies investigating the genetic factors in the development of PAD include family and twin studies, gene studies and ankle-brachial index (ABI) variance analysis [23-25]. Some studies have found that 20 to 50 percent of the variance in ABI can be explained by genetic factors [18, 23, 26]. However, another study on twins found that traditional cardiovascular risk factors were significantly more common in twins with PAD compared to those without PAD. Concordances and correlations were higher in monozygotic compared with dizygotic twins, suggesting genetic influences in PAD [24]. Despite finding such correlations, a study found no significant difference in the prevalence of PAD between dizygotic and monozygotic twins [23]. A case control study found that a family history of PAD was present significantly more often in patients with PAD than in controls even after adjusting for conventional risk factors. The association was stronger in younger subjects (age <68 years), and a greater number of affected relatives with PAD was also more strongly associated with PAD [27]. A meta-analysis of possible genetic susceptibility to PAD found no strong supportive evidence for most genetic polymorphisms but did identify three genes that may be important variants [28]. The role of the physician can be listed as giving importance to family history and being aware of early onset atherosclerosis in the family.

Smoking

Smoking is a risk factor for PAD promoting endothelial dysfunction, and altering lipid metabolism and coagulation [29]. The risk is higher for PAD than for Coronary Artery Disease (CAD). The PAD risk increases in current heavier smokers, and the number of cigarettes is much more. In a systematic review that included North America, South America, Europe, Australia, and Africa assessed the magnitude of increased risk of PAD in current smokers relative to never smokers (OR 2.71, 95% CI 2.28-3.21), and ex-smokers relative to never smokers (OR 1.67, 95% CI 1.43-1.81) [30]. Smoking has harmful effects on PAD and all body systems. It can impair cardiac autonomic modulation in patients with symptomatic PAD [31]. Smoking is associated with an increased risk of incident intermittent claudication and decline in ABI compared with other risk factors [32, 33]. Smoking is also associated with lower levels of subcutaneous collagen. The scarcity of collagen tissue significantly reduces cutaneous microvascular function and promotes an environment conducive to PAD-associated ischemic ulcerations. However, wound healing rates in limb ischemia were found to be low in active smokers; yet no link was found between the amount smoked and outcomes [34, 35]. Because there is insufficient evidence for risk stratification, all active smokers should be encouraged to quit smoking, and elective intervention among smokers with cladicatio should be delayed until patients greatly reduce their smoking [36].

A significant relationship between cigarette dose and risk for PAD has been reported [37]. A greater number of pack-years of smoking is also associated with increasing disease severity, negative effects on the patency of vascular reconstruction, and an increased risk of amputation and cardiovascular mortality following revascularization [38]. However, heavier smokers are more likely to develop peripheral artery disease than light smokers and that former smokers have a persistently increased risk compared with never smokers [39]. Some studies have shown that the risk is linked to gender and is higher in women. These situations pose a significant gender-related health burden and pose a particular challenge for managing this risk factor among women. For example, gender-related motivations for starting tobacco use should be taken into account when designing smoking cessation campaigns [40].

Interventions about smoking are very important in primary care. Although warnings about smoking cessation increase patients' admission to smoking cessation clinics, many of these patients quickly relapse and 72% of all patients smoking at baseline are still smoking at 12 months. Better strategies are needed to provide continuous cessation support [41, 42]. The guidelines incorporate patient behavioral change and the "Five A's": Ask, Advise, Assess, Assist and Arrange. Patients with PAD who smoke cigarettes or use other forms of tobacco should be advised at every visit to quit. Patients with PAD who smoke cigarettes should be assisted in developing a plan for quitting that includes pharmacotherapy (ie, varenicline, bupropion, and/or nicotine replacement therapy) and/or referral to a smoking cessation program [4]. Pharmacotherapeutic tools, including nicotine replacement therapies and non-nicotine therapies are considered. Complete and permanent cessation of smoking is by far the single most important factor determining the outcome of patients with intermittent claudication [43].

Nicotine replacement treatment approximately doubles the cessation rate in unselected smokers. Bupropion and Varenicline has a similar benefit when used with intensive support. Both treatments are now available on prescription, and every patient with claudication should be offered nicotine replacement treatment in the first place. Not all nicotine replacement preparations are the same, and if one preparation fails then other preparations, or combinations with different delivery profiles, should be tried [44]. The Cochrane group found smoking classes but not alternative therapies to be beneficial [45-47]. Smoking cessation and exercise are considered the two most important treatments for PAD [48]. Patients with PAD should also avoid exposure to environmental tobacco smoke at work, at home, and in public places if they are not smokers [4].

Diabetes

The TASC II guidelines conclude that, for all patients with diabetes, the relative risk of developing peripheral artery disease is similar that of people who smoke [49]. Poor glycemic control is associated with an increased risk of PAD [7]. A prospective cohort study with more than 20 years follow-up found an increased risk of death (HR 2.9, 95% CI 1.3-4.0) for patients with diabetes and PAD, compared with those without diabetes [50]. Diabetes is equivalent to the risk of a coronary artery disease, and the risk of developing PAD depends on the severity and duration of the disease. Patients with diabetes are likely to have more advanced artery disease at initial diagnosis and have worse outcomes than non-diabetic patients [50, 51]. Patients with diabetes are more likely to be asymptomatic because of the co-existence of neuropathy in a substantial proportion. Peripheral artery disease in this population is more likely to be found in more distal vessels in the calf. Infection and neuropathy are also contributing factors, although the severity of PAD increases the risk of amputation in these patients. In the Veterans Aging Cohort Study, the presence of neuropathy or retinopathy caused by microvascular diseased significantly increased the risk of amputation (relative risk 3.7, 95% CI 3.0-4.6). PAD alone had a 13.9-fold increased risk of amputation, and a combination of PAD and microvascular disease was associated with a 22.7-fold increase. Microvascular disease was also associated with more distal amputations [53]. Population studies have found that around half of patients with a diabetic foot ulcer have peripheral artery disease [54].

While alcohol consumption has typically been associated with a protective effect on vessels, one review found that heavy alcohol use in patients with type II diabetes was associated with an increased risk for lower extremity PAD (OR 6.25, 95% CI 1.78-22.65) [55]. A dose-response relationship was also found between prolonged alcohol consumption and PAD [54].

Diagnosis or exclusion of type 2 diabetes is important in patients with peripheral arterial disease, but this is not straightforward [56]. A threshold of fasting glucose >126mg/dl, the oral glucose tolerance test is the "gold standard" to diagnose but it is logistically difficult to perform. In practice, random blood glucose may be the easiest measure to obtain; a random blood glucose >200 mg/dl (plasma glucose performed in an accredited laboratory not finger prick, capillary glucose should be evaluated) is diagnostic of type 2 diabetes, and a random blood glucose of 126-200mg/dl should be followed with an oral glucose tolerance test (Table 3) [57].

Table 3. Plasma glucose and A1C levels

	Fasting Plasma Glucose	Plasma Glucose in Oral Glucose Tolerance Test	A1C
Normal	<100 mg/dL or 5.5 mmol/L	<140 mg/dL or 7.8 mmol/L	<5.7% or 39 mmol/mol
Pre-Diabetes	≥100 mg/dL or 5.5 mmol/L	≥140 mg/dL or 7.8 mmol/L	≥5.7% or 39 mmol/mol
Diabetes	≥126 mg/dL or 7.0 mmol/L	≥200 mg/dL or 11.1 mmol/L	≥6.5% or 48 mmol/mol

However, it is important to follow up diabetes in patients with PAD. Providing glycemic control in patients with diabetes and PAD, keeping A1C (<7.0%) at optimum values, providing life-style changes are valuable in terms of preventing complications due to PAD. AHA emphasize that glycemic control can be beneficial for patients with intermittent claudication to reduce limb-related outcomes. Management of diabetes mellitus in the patient with PAD should be coordinated between members of the healthcare team [4]. Nutrition is a key factor in the management of diabetes for normoglycemic control as well as medication. Medical nutrition for people with diabetes should be personalized, taking into account their usual food and eating habits, metabolic profiles, treatment goals and desired results. Diabetic patients' diets are based on proper carbohydrate, protein, fat and calorie intake. Foods containing whole grains, fruits, vegetables, and low-fat dairy carbohydrates should be included in a healthy diet. Regarding the glycemic effects of carbohydrates, the total amount of carbohydrates present in meals or snacks is more important than the source or type. Since sucrose does not increase glycemia more than isocaloric amounts, foods containing starch, sucrose and sucrose need not be restricted by people with diabetes; however, they should be substituted with other carbohydrate sources or, if added, turned off with insulin or other glucose-lowering drugs. Non-nutritious sweeteners are safe when consumed within acceptable daily intake levels. The effects of protein on regulation of energy intake, satiety and long-term weight loss have not been studied enough. The long-term efficacy and safety of high protein low carbohydrate diets are unknown. In patients with controlled type 2 diabetes, protein ingested does not increase plasma glucose concentrations, although protein is as strong an insulin secretion stimulator as carbohydrate. For patients with diabetes, especially those who are not in optimal glucose control, protein requirements may be greater, but not greater than normal intake. Less than 10% of the energy intake in the diet of diabetic patients should be obtained from saturated fat. Some patients (i.e., people with LDL cholesterol ≥100 mg/dl) may benefit from lowering their saturated fat intake to <7% of their energy intake. Dietary cholesterol intake should be <300 mg/day. Some patients (i.e., people with LDL cholesterol ≥100 mg/dl) may benefit from lowering dietary cholesterol to <200 mg/day. Structured programs that emphasize lifestyle changes, including training, reduced fat (<30% of daily energy) and energy intake, regular physical activity, and regular participant contact can result in 5-7% long-term weight loss, starting weight. Exercise and behavior modification are most helpful in addition to other weight loss strategies. Exercise is helpful in maintaining weight loss. Standard weight reduction diets are unlikely to result in long-term weight loss when used alone. Structured intensive lifestyle programs are required [58].

Pre-diabetes can be defined as a gray zone between normal and diabetic plasma glucose levels. Patients with pre-diabetes can be converted to normoglycemia with easy and simple interventions in lifestyle changes. Moreover, long-term studies have shown that the risk of progress from pre-diabetes to diabetes can be extended for 10 years with adoption to the healthy lifestyle changes. It is stated that one third of patients with pre-diabetes can develop diabetes within 4 years if left untreated. The number of pre-diabetic patients who develop diabetes can be reduced to 20% with healthy lifestyle interventions [59]. Raising awareness of individuals with pre-diabetes and categorizing of risk can help primary care physicians to understand potential interventions that could help reduce the number of patients who will develop diabetes. Intervention to prevent diabetes development by identifying pre-diabetic individuals is crucial to our efforts to make healthcare more cost-effective and save lives. Studies have shown that it is possible to prevent the progression of pre-diabetes to diabetes and to convert pre-diabetes to a normal glucose level. In addition, pre-diabetes and diabetes complications can only be prevented by achieving a normal glucose pattern [60]. Pre-diabetes is a critical stage because it is reversible and could serve as a potential pathway combating diabetes. Pre-diabetes does not increase the risk of microvascular disease like diabetes, the main risk in this condition being diabetes, making it important to act before encountering major morbidities due to diabetes. It should be kept in mind that the primary goal of healthy lifestyle interventions in this area is to prevent diabetes and its complications [61]. For individuals without diabetes, fasting blood glucose level is moderately and non-linearly associated with risk of vascular disease [62].

Dyslipidemia

Patients with PAD are more likely to have dyslipidemia which is defined as increased levels of triglycerides and/or cholesterol, lipoprotein (a), apolipoprotein B, and very low-density lipoprotein. Conversely, the "protective" lipoproteins such as high-density lipoprotein (HDL) cholesterol and apolipoprotein A-I and A-II levels, are low [63]. In the Doctors' Health Study, the ratio of total cholesterol to HDL cholesterol was the best independent predictor of PAD [64]. Lipoprotein (a) is genetically determined and controlled by a single gene locus and also a significant independent risk factor for PAD. The risk of intermittent claudication is high in patients with higher levels of plasma lipoprotein (a) [65].

Treatment for hyperlipidemia can reduce the risk of progression of PAD and the incidence of intermittent claudication. A heart protection study showed that lowering total cholesterol and low-density lipoprotein cholesterol by 25% with a statin reduced cardiovascular mortality and morbidity in patients with peripheral artery disease [66]. Any patient with peripheral artery disease should be treated with a statin. The lipid profile should be measured before starting treatment and six weeks after initiation to check the reduction in cholesterol and identify patients with very high cholesterol concentrations or hypertriglyceridemia to refer for further investigation [57]. Lifestyle recommendations addressing physical activity, medical nutrition therapy, and smoking cessation are also recommended. The level of physical activity needed for a beneficial impact on risk remains controversial. However, physical activity should include moderate-intensity aerobic activity (4 to 7 kcal/min) four to six times per week as a 30-minute single session or as multiple sessions of at least 10 minutes at a time. Muscle strengthening activity should be performed two times per week. This level of activity is well tolerated by most middle-aged or older patients. However, people who are initially unfit or sedentary should start at lower intensity. Nevertheless, it could be strongly suggested that even low levels of physical activity may modify the status of the patients [67]. Medical nutrition therapy should focus on a reduced-calorie diet that includes more than five servings a day of fruits and vegetables, whole grains, fish and lean meats, limited saturated and trans fats, 2 g/day of plant stanols, and 10 to 25 g/day of fiber [68].

When goals have been achieved, lipid status should be monitored every 6 to 12 months depending on adherence and consistency in results. Situations that warrant more frequent monitoring include deterioration of diabetes control, change in medication or medical condition predisposing to secondary dyslipidemia, new risk factor, or as new evidence emerges. Consultation to a certified lipid specialist or an endocrinologist is recommended for patients with lipid abnormalities on intensive treatment, when type 2 diabetes and dyslipidemia coexist, or if atherothrombotic disease progresses despite favorable lipid levels [69].

Hypertension

High blood pressure increases the risk of intermittent claudication, the most common symptom of PAD. Hypertension is strongly associated with the development of atherosclerosis in males and females [70]. Those with hypertension have a higher risk of developing PAD symptoms, such as intermittent claudication [71]. On the other hand, the NHANES study found that hypertensive patients had an even higher prevalence of asymptomatic PAD [7]. The association between hypertension and PAD among patients older than 60 years of age was particularly strong in those with untreated or poorly controlled [72]. For other patients with PAD, they are less likely to receive antihypertensive therapy than those with other cardiovascular disease [7].

The benefit of treating hypertension in reducing stroke and coronary events is well recognized. The data show a target of less than 140/85 mm Hg for non-diabetic patients and less than 140/80 mm Hg for patients with type 2 diabetes [73]. However, the evidence for various anti-hypertensive drug classes in PAD is poor, so that it is unknown whether significant benefit or risk accrues from their use [74]. Ramipril, an angiotensin converting enzyme inhibitor, reduces cardiovascular morbidity and mortality by approximately 25% in patients with peripheral artery disease [75]. The implication of the heart outcomes prevention evaluation study is that most patients with peripheral artery disease would benefit from an angiotensin converting enzyme inhibitor provided that the treatment is not associated with impaired renal function due to occult renal artery stenosis [57].

Non-pharmacological methods that significantly reduce blood pressure (BP) are limiting alcohol consumption, increasing exercise, weight loss, recreational activities, reduce salt intake, and dietary approaches to stop hypertension (DASH) diet (Table 4) [76]. The DASH diet is a lifelong approach to healthy eating, designed to help treat or prevent high blood pressure. The DASH diet plan was developed to reduce drug-free blood pressure in research supported by the National Institutes of Health [77]. It encourages patients to eat a variety of foods rich in nutrients that help reduce sodium in their diet and lower blood pressure, such as potassium, calcium, and magnesium. By following the DASH diet, patients can reduce their blood pressure by a few points in few weeks. Over time, the most patient blood pressure (systolic blood pressure) may drop by 2 to 14 points, which can make a significant difference in health risks. As the DASH diet is a healthy diet, it provides health benefits as well as lowering blood pressure. The DASH diet also complies with dietary recommendations to prevent osteoporosis, cancer, heart disease, stroke, and diabetes. The DASH diet emphasizes vegetables, fruits and low-fat dairy products, and moderate amounts of whole grains, fish, poultry and nuts. The standard DASH diet meets the recommendation of the Dietary Guidelines for Americans to keep sodium intake below 2,300 mg per day [78].

**Table 4. Nonpharmacological measures
and their estimated reduce in BP**

Nonpharmacological measures	Estimated reduce in BP
Body weight reduction	10 kg loss in body weight reduces BP 5-20 mmHg
DASH diet	2-14mmHg
Cut salt	2-8 mmHg
Exercise	4-9 mmHg
Low alcohol intake	2-4 mmHg

The American Heart Association recommends 1,500 mg of sodium per day as an upper limit for all adults. The foods at the core of the DASH diet are naturally low in sodium. Using sodium-free spices, not adding salt when cooking rice, pasta or hot cereal, rinsing canned foods to remove some of the sodium, buying foods labeled "no salt added," "sodium-free," "low sodium" or "very low sodium" can be tips for using low sodium. One teaspoon of table salt has 2,325 mg of sodium. Even low-fat soups, canned vegetables, ready-to-eat cereals and sliced turkey from the local deli have lots of sodium [77].

In addition, grains should be taken 6 to 8 servings a day. Grains includes bread, cereal, rice and pasta. Whole grains contain more fiber and nutrients than refined grains. Grains are naturally low in fat. Vegetables should be taken 4-5 servings a day. Tomatoes, carrots, broccoli, sweet potatoes, greens, and other vegetables are available with fiber, vitamins, and minerals such as potassium and magnesium. Fruits should be taken in 4-5 portions a day. Like vegetables, they contain fiber, potassium, and magnesium and are typically low in fat. Dairy products should be taken 2-3 servings a day. Milk, yogurt, cheese, and other dairy products are major sources of calcium, vitamin D, and protein. However, low-fat or non-fat dairy products should be preferred because otherwise they can be a great source of fat and many are saturated. Lean meats, poultry and fish should be ingested about 200g or less per day. Meat can be a rich source of protein, B vitamins, iron and zinc. Cutting meat portions will provide room for more vegetables. Eating heart-friendly fish such as salmon, herring, and tuna is a good option. These types of fish are high in omega-3 fatty acids that are healthy for the patient's heart. Nuts, seeds and legumes should be taken in 4-5 servings per week. Almonds, sunflower seeds, kidney beans, peas, lentils, and other foods in this family are good sources of magnesium, potassium, and protein. They are also full of fiber and phytochemicals, plant compounds that can protect against some cancers and cardiovascular diseases. Portion sizes are small and intended to be consumed only a few times a week because these foods are higher in calories. Fats and oils should be taken 2 to 3 servings a day. The oil helps the body absorb essential vitamins and helps the immune system. However, too much fat increases the risk of heart disease, diabetes and obesity. The DASH diet seeks to maintain a healthy balance by focusing on healthier monounsaturated fats, limiting total fat to less than 30 percent of daily calories from fat. Desserts should be taken 5 servings or less per week. When following the DASH diet, it is not necessary to ban sweets completely. While the DASH diet is not a weight-loss program, patients may indeed lose weight because it can help them guide toward healthier food choices. The DASH diet generally includes about 2,000 calories a day.

Drinking too much alcohol can increase blood pressure. The Dietary Guidelines for Americans recommends that men limit alcohol to no more than two drinks a day and women to one or less. The DASH diet doesn't address caffeine consumption. The influence of caffeine on blood pressure remains unclear. But caffeine can cause blood pressure to rise at least temporarily [78].

CONCLUSION

Primary care is the principal target for investigation if the aim is improved population-based care. Family physicians play a key role, as they are the first point of contact for recognition, diagnosis and referral. The role of the family physician is particularly important in the prevention and early recognition of PAD. The complex approach of our method allows the practitioner to identify at-risk patients belonging to the turbid region. In the long term, initiating a complex screening program at the primary care level significantly improves both patients' quality of life and life expectancy by facilitating the diagnosis of patients with PAD, leading to earlier treatment initiation [79]. Considering all these risk factors in the population, family physicians have also a crucial role to arise PAD awareness among patients and general population. Increased awareness could enable earlier, appropriate and effective management of PAD and adherence to secondary prevention strategies for the modification of PAD risk factors at primary health care settings. Inquiring about the patient's education about PAD symptoms and risks and exercise tolerance can address the issue of under-reporting. Annual reviews can provide an opportunity to investigate PAD symptoms and highlight those that require further investigation. Given better information when diagnosed with PAD and the tendency of patients to tolerate worsening symptoms, it is appropriate to initiate annual follow-up. The medical approach to peripheral artery disease is multifaceted and includes cholesterol reduction, antiplatelet therapy, anticoagulation, peripheral vasodilators, blood pressure management, exercise therapy, and smoking cessation. Adherence to this regimen may reduce limb-related complications such as critical limb ischemia and amputation, as well as systemic complications of atherosclerosis such as stroke and myocardial infarction. The effect of treatment has traditionally focused on outcomes such as primary patency and limb salvage, but quality of life (QOL) is considered an important additional primary endpoint in a more patient-focused healthcare system. To take patients individual opinions more into account, it is necessary to focus on quality-of-life research to determine superior therapy in patients with PAD [80-82]. Documenting the distance walked until onset of symptoms allows progression of the disease to be monitored. Intervention is unnecessary if there is no impairment in quality of life, but risk factor identification and management must take place. Evidence from large population studies have found less than half of these patients have adequate risk factor modification by time of referral [83-85].

REFERENCES

[1]   Fowkes, F. G., Rudan, D., Rudan, I., Aboyans, V., Denenberg, J. O., McDermott, M. M., Norman, P. E., Sampson, U. K., Williams, L. J., Mensah, G. A., & Criqui, M. H. (2013). Comparison of global estimates of prevalence and risk factors for peripheral artery disease in 2000 and 2010: a systematic review and analysis. *Lancet (London, England)*, *382*(9901), 1329–1340. https://doi.org/10.1016/S0140-6736(13)61249-0.

[2]   Tunstall-Pedoe, H., Peters, S., Woodward, M., Struthers, A. D., & Belch, J. (2017). Twenty-Year Predictors of Peripheral Arterial Disease Compared With Coronary Heart Disease in the Scottish Heart Health Extended Cohort (SHHEC). *Journal of the American*

Heart Association, *6*(9), e005967. https://doi.org/10.1161/JAHA.117. 005967.

[3] Fowkes, F. G., Aboyans, V., Fowkes, F. J., McDermott, M. M., Sampson, U. K., & Criqui, M. H. (2017). Peripheral artery disease: epidemiology and global perspectives. *Nature reviews. Cardiology*, *14*(3), 156–170. https://doi.org/10.1038/nrcardio.2016.179.

[4] Gerhard-Herman, M. D., Gornik, H. L., Barrett, C., Barshes, N. R., Corriere, M. A., Drachman, D. E., Fleisher, L. A., Fowkes, F., Hamburg, N. M., Kinlay, S., Lookstein, R., Misra, S., Mureebe, L., Olin, J. W., Patel, R., Regensteiner, J. G., Schanzer, A., Shishehbor, M. H., Stewart, K. J., Treat-Jacobson, D., ... Walsh, M. E. (2017). 2016 AHA/ACC Guideline on the Management of Patients With Lower Extremity Peripheral Artery Disease: Executive Summary: A Report of the American College of Cardiology/American Heart Association Task Force on Clinical Practice Guidelines. *Journal of the American College of Cardiology*, *69*(11), 1465–1508. https://doi.org/10.1016/j.jacc.2016.11.008.

[5] Feringa, H. H., Bax, J. J., Hoeks, S., van Waning, V. H., Elhendy, A., Karagiannis, S., Vidakovic, R., Schouten, O., Boersma, E., & Poldermans, D. (2007). A prognostic risk index for long-term mortality in patients with peripheral arterial disease. *Archives of internal medicine*, *167*(22), 2482–2489. https://doi.org/10.1001/ archinte.167.22.2482.

[6] Kröger, K., Stang, A., Kondratieva, J., Moebus, S., Beck, E., Schmermund, A., Möhlenkamp, S., Dragano, N., Siegrist, J., Jöckel, K. H., Erbel, R., & Heinz Nixdorf Recall Study Group (2006). Prevalence of peripheral arterial disease - results of the Heinz Nixdorf recall study. *European journal of epidemiology*, *21*(4), 279–285. https://doi.org/10.1007/s10654-006-0015-9.

[7] Selvin, E., & Erlinger, T. P. (2004). Prevalence of and risk factors for peripheral arterial disease in the United States: results from the National Health and Nutrition Examination Survey, 1999-2000. *Circulation*, *110*(6), 738–743. https://doi.org/10.1161/01.CIR.000013 7913.26087.F0.

[8]   Savji, N., Rockman, C. B, Skolnick, A. H., Guo, Y., Adelman, M.A., Riles, T., & Berger, J. S. (2013). Association between advanced age and vascular disease in different arterial territories: a population database of over 3.6 million subjects. *J Am Coll Cardiol*, 61(16), 1736.

[9]   Hylton, J. R., Smith, C. A., Li, C. S., & Pevec, W. C. (2014). Octogenarians develop infrapopliteal arterial occlusive disease in the absence of traditional risk factors. *Annals of vascular surgery*, 28(7), 1712–1718. https://doi.org/10.1016/j.avsg.2014.04.005.

[10]   Song, P., Rudan, D., Zhu, Y., Fowkes, F., Rahimi, K., Fowkes, F., & Rudan, I. (2019). Global, regional, and national prevalence and risk factors for peripheral artery disease in 2015: an updated systematic review and analysis. *The Lancet. Global health*, 7(8), e1020–e1030. https://doi.org/10.1016/S2214-109X(19)30255-4.

[11]   Hirsch, A. T., Allison, M. A., Gomes, A. S., Corriere, M. A., Duval, S., Ershow, A. G., Hiatt, W. R., Karas, R. H., Lovell, M. B., McDermott, M. M., Mendes, D. M., Nussmeier, N. A., Treat-Jacobson, D., American Heart Association Council on Peripheral Vascular Disease, Council on Cardiovascular Nursing, Council on Cardiovascular Radiology and Intervention, Council on Cardiovascular Surgery and Anesthesia, Council on Clinical Cardiology, & Council on Epidemiology and Prevention (2012). A call to action: women and peripheral artery disease: a scientific statement from the American Heart Association. *Circulation*, 125(11), 1449–1472. https://doi.org/10.1161/CIR.0b013e31824c39ba.

[12]   Brevetti, G., Bucur, R., Balbarini, A., Melillo, E., Novo, S., Muratori, I., & Chiariello, M. (2008). Women and peripheral arterial disease: same disease, different issues. *Journal of cardiovascular medicine (Hagerstown, Md.)*, 9(4), 382–388.

[13]   Hiramoto, J. S., Katz, R., Weisman, S., & Conte, M. (2014). Gender-specific risk factors for peripheral artery disease in a voluntary screening population. *Journal of the American Heart Association*, 3(2), e000651. https://doi.org/10.1161/JAHA.113.000651.

[14] Sigvant, B., Wiberg-Hedman, K., Bergqvist, D., Rolandsson, O., Andersson, B., Persson, E., & Wahlberg, E. (2007). A population-based study of peripheral arterial disease prevalence with special focus on critical limb ischemia and sex differences. *J Vasc Surg*, 45(6),1185.

[15] George, J., Rapsomaniki, E., Pujades-Rodriguez, M., Shah, A. D., Denaxas, S., Herrett, E., Smeeth, L., Timmis, A., & Hemingway, H. (2015). How Does Cardiovascular Disease First Present in Women and Men? Incidence of 12 Cardiovascular Diseases in a Contemporary Cohort of 1,937,360 People. *Circulation*, *132*(14), 1320–1328. https://doi.org/10.1161/CIRCULATIONAHA.114.013 797.

[16] Rockman, C. B., Maldonado, T. S., Jacobowitz, G. R., Adelman, M. A., & Riles, T. S. (2012). Hormone replacement therapy is associated with a decreased prevalence of peripheral arterial disease in postmenopausal women. *Annals of Vascular Surgery*, Apr,26(3),411-418. doi: 10.1016/j.avsg.2011.10.012.

[17] Allison, M. A., Cushman, M., Solomon, C., Aboyans, V., McDermott, M. M., Goff, D. C., Jr, & Criqui, M. H. (2009). Ethnicity and risk factors for change in the ankle-brachial index: the Multi-Ethnic Study of Atherosclerosis. *Journal of vascular surgery*, *50*(5), 1049–1056. https://doi.org/10.1016/j.jvs.2009.05.061.

[18] Kullo, I. J., Bailey, K. R., Kardia, S. L., Mosley, T. H., Jr, Boerwinkle, E., & Turner, S. T. (2003). Ethnic differences in peripheral arterial disease in the NHLBI Genetic Epidemiology Network of Arteriopathy (GENOA) study. *Vascular medicine (London, England)*, *8*(4), 237–242. https://doi.org/10.1191/1358863x 03vm511oa.

[19] Meadows, T. A., Bhatt, D. L., Hirsch, A. T., Creager, M. A., Califf, R. M., Ohman, E. M., Cannon, C. P., Eagle, K. A., Alberts, M. J., Goto, S., Smith, S. C. Jr., Wilson, P. W., Watson, K. E., Steg, P. G., REACH Registry Investigators. (2009). Ethnic differences in the prevalence and treatment of cardiovascular risk factors in US outpatients with peripheral arterial disease: insights from the

reduction of atherothrombosis for continued health (REACH) registry. *Am Heart J*, 158(6),1038.

[20] Subramaniam, T., Nang, E. E., Lim, S. C., Wu, Y., Khoo, C. M., Lee, J., Heng, D., Chew, S. K., Wong, T. Y., & Tai, E. S. (2011). Distribution of ankle-brachial index and the risk factors of peripheral artery disease in a multi-ethnic Asian population. *Vascular medicine (London, England)*, *16*(2), 87–95. https://doi.org/10.1177/ 1358863X11400781.

[21] Sebastianski, M., Makowsky, M. J., Dorgan, M., & Tsuyuki, R. T. (2014). Paradoxically lower prevalence of peripheral arterial disease in South Asians: a systematic review and meta-analysis. *Heart (British Cardiac Society)*, *100*(2), 100–105. https://doi.org/10.1136/ heartjnl-2013-303605.

[22] Leeper, N. J., Kullo, I. J., & Cooke, J. P. (2012). Genetics of peripheral artery disease. *Circulation*, *125*(25), 3220–3228. https://doi.org/10.1161/CIRCULATIONAHA.111.033878.

[23] Carmelli, D., Fabsitz, R. R., Swan, G. E., Reed, T., Miller, B., & Wolf, P. A. (2000). Contribution of genetic and environmental influences to ankle-brachial blood pressure index in the NHLBI Twin Study. National Heart, Lung, and Blood Institute. *American journal of epidemiology*, *151*(5), 452–458. https://doi.org/10.1093/oxford journals.aje.a010230.

[24] Wahlgren, C. M., & Magnusson, P. K. (2011). Genetic influences on peripheral arterial disease in a twin population. *Arteriosclerosis, thrombosis, and vascular biology*, *31*(3), 678–682. https://doi.org/10. 1161/ATVBAHA.110.210385.

[25] Allison, M. A., Peralta, C. A., Wassel, C. L., Aboyans, V., Arnett, D. K., Cushman, M., Eng, J., Ix, J., Rich, S. S., & Criqui, M. H. (2010). Genetic ancestry and lower extremity peripheral artery disease in the Multi-Ethnic Study of Atherosclerosis. *Vascular medicine (London, England)*, *15*(5), 351–359. https://doi.org/10.1177/1358863X103 75586.

[26] Murabito, J. M., Guo, C. Y., Fox, C. S., & D'Agostino, R. B. (2006). Heritability of the ankle-brachial index: the Framingham Offspring

study. *American journal of epidemiology*, *164*(10), 963–968. https://doi.org/10.1093/aje/kwj295.

[27] Khaleghi, M., Isseh, I. N., Bailey, K. R., & Kullo, I. J. (2014). Family history as a risk factor for peripheral arterial disease. *The American journal of cardiology*, *114*(6), 928–932. https://doi.org/10.1016/j.amjcard.2014.06.029.

[28] Zintzaras, E., & Zdoukopoulos, N. (2009). A field synopsis and meta-analysis of genetic association studies in peripheral arterial disease: The CUMAGAS-PAD database. *American journal of epidemiology*, *170*(1), 1–11. https://doi.org/10.1093/aje/kwp094.

[29] Lu, J. T., & Creager, M. A. (2004). The relationship of cigarette smoking to peripheral arterial disease. *Reviews in cardiovascular medicine*, *5*(4), 189–193.

[30] Lu, L., Mackay, D. F., & Pell, J. P. (2014). Meta-analysis of the association between cigarette smoking and peripheral arterial disease. *Heart (British Cardiac Society)*, *100*(5), 414–423. https://doi.org/10.1136/heartjnl-2013-304082.

[31] Quintella Farah, B., Silva Rigoni, V. L., de Almeida Correia, M., Wolosker, N., Puech-Leao, P., Grizzo Cucato, G., & Ritti-Dias, R. M. (2019). Influence of smoking on physical function, physical activity, and cardiovascular health parameters in patients with symptomatic peripheral arterial disease: A cross-sectional study. *Journal of vascular nursing: official publication of the Society for Peripheral Vascular Nursing*, *37*(2), 106–112. https://doi.org/10.1016/j.jvn.2019.01.003.

[32] Kollerits, B., Heinrich, J., Pichler, M., Rantner, B., Klein-Weigel, P., Wölke, G., Brasche, S., Strube, G., Kronenberg, F., & Erfurt Male Cohort (2008). Intermittent claudication in the Erfurt Male Cohort (ERFORT) Study: its determinants and the impact on mortality. A population-based prospective cohort study with 30 years of follow-up. *Atherosclerosis*, *198*(1), 214–222. https://doi.org/10.1016/j.atherosclerosis.2007.09.012.

[33] Aboyans, V., Criqui, M. H., Denenberg, J. O., Knoke, J. D., Ridker, P. M., & Fronek, A. (2006). Risk factors for progression of

peripheral arterial disease in large and small vessels. *Circulation*, *113*(22), 2623–2629. https://doi.org/10.1161/CIRCULATIONAHA. 105.608679.

[34] Kokkinidis, D. G., Giannopoulos, S., Haider, M., Jordan, T., Sarkar, A., Singh, G. D., Secemsky, E. A., Giri, J., Beckman, J. A., & Armstrong, E. J. (2020). Active smoking is associated with higher rates of incomplete wound healing after endovascular treatment of critical limb ischemia. *Vascular medicine (London, England)*, *25*(5), 427–435. https://doi.org/10.1177/1358863X20916526.

[35] Schlieder, I., Richard, M., Nacar, A., Rieger, R., Bethge, A., Vijayakumar, S., & Dietzek, A. M. (2019). Active Tobacco Use in Patients with Claudication Does Not Affect Outcomes after Endovascular Interventions. *Annals of vascular surgery*, *60*, 279–285. https://doi.org/10.1016/j.avsg.2019.02.016.

[36] Weissler, E. H., Gutierrez, J. A., Patel, M. R., & Swaminathan, R. V. (2021). Successful Peripheral Vascular Intervention in Patients with High-risk Comorbidities or Lesion Characteristics. *Current cardiology reports*, *23*(4), 32. https://doi.org/10.1007/s11886-021-01465-8.

[37] Hirsch, A. T., Criqui, M. H., Treat-Jacobson, D., Regensteiner, J. G., Creager, M. A., Olin, J. W., Krook, S. H., Hunninghake, D. B., Comerota, A. J., Walsh, M. E., McDermott, M. M., & Hiatt, W. R. (2001). Peripheral arterial disease detection, awareness, and treatment in primary care. *JAMA*, *286*(11), 1317–1324. https://doi.org/10.1001/jama.286.11.1317.

[38] Fanka W. B., Chaney S. (2019) Tobacco Education: Reduced Risk for Peripheral Artery Disease. *Intern Med* 9:303.

[39] Willigendael, E. M., Teijink, J. A., Bartelink, M. L., Kuiken, B. W., Boiten, J., Moll, F. L., Büller, H. R., & Prins, M. H. (2004). Influence of smoking on incidence and prevalence of peripheral arterial disease. *Journal of vascular surgery*, *40*(6), 1158–1165. https://doi.org/10.1016/j.jvs.2004.08.049.

[40] Barochiner, J., Aparicio, L. S., & Waisman, G. D. (2014). Challenges associated with peripheral arterial disease in women. *Vascular health*

and risk management, *10*, 115–128. https://doi.org/10.2147/ VHRM.S45181.

[41] Smith, B. K., Adsit, R. T., Jorenby, D. E., Matsumura, J. S., & Fiore, M. C. (2015). Utilization of the Electronic Health Record to Improve Provision of Smoking Cessation Resources for Vascular Surgery Inpatients. *International journal of cardiovascular research*, *4*(5), 10.4172/2324-8602.1000231. https://doi.org/10.4172/2324-8602.100 0231.

[42] Patel, K. K., Jones, P. G., Ellerbeck, E. F., Buchanan, D. M., Chan, P. S., Pacheco, C. M., Moneta, G., Spertus, J. A., & Smolderen, K. G. (2018). Underutilization of Evidence-Based Smoking Cessation Support Strategies Despite High Smoking Addiction Burden in Peripheral Artery Disease Specialty Care: Insights from the International PORTRAIT Registry. *Journal of the American Heart Association*, *7*(20), e010076. https://doi.org/10.1161/JAHA.118. 010076.

[43] Davies, A. (2000). The practical management of claudication. *BMJ (Clinical research ed.)*, *321*(7266), 911–912. https://doi.org/10.1136/ bmj.321.7266.911.

[44] Anczak, J. D., & Nogler, R. A., 2nd (2003). Tobacco cessation in primary care: maximizing intervention strategies. *Clinical medicine & research*, *1*(3), 201–216. https://doi.org/10.3121/cmr.1.3.201.

[45] Abbot, N. C., Stead, L. F., White, A. R., Barnes, J., & Ernst, E. (2000). Hypnotherapy for smoking cessation. *The Cochrane database of systematic reviews*, (2), CD001008. https://doi.org/10. 1002/14651858.CD001008.

[46] Hajek, P., & Stead, L. F. (2000). Aversive smoking for smoking cessation. *The Cochrane database of systematic reviews*, (2), CD000546. https://doi.org/10.1002/14651858.CD000546.

[47] White, A. R., Rampes, H., & Ernst, E. (2000). Acupuncture for smoking cessation. *The Cochrane database of systematic reviews*, (2), CD000009. https://doi.org/10.1002/14651858.CD000009.

[48] Mukherjee, D., & Yadav, J. S. (2001). Update on peripheral vascular diseases: from smoking cessation to stenting. *Cleveland Clinic*

journal of medicine, *68*(8), 723–733. https://doi.org/10.3949/ccjm. 68.8.723.

[49] Norgren, L., Hiatt, W. R., Dormandy, J. A., Nehler, M. R., Harris, K. A., Fowkes, F. G., & TASC II Working Group (2007). Inter-Society Consensus for the Management of Peripheral Arterial Disease (TASC II). *Journal of vascular surgery*, 45 Suppl S, S5–S67. https://doi.org/ 10.1016/j.jvs.2006.12.037.

[50] Leibson, C. L., Ransom, J. E., Olson, W., Zimmerman, B. R., O'fallon, W. M., & Palumbo, P. J. (2004). Peripheral arterial disease, diabetes, and mortality. *Diabetes care*, *27*(12), 2843–2849. https://doi.org/10.2337/diacare.27.12.2843.

[51] Jude, E. B., Oyibo, S. O., Chalmers, N., & Boulton, A. J. (2001). Peripheral arterial disease in diabetic and nondiabetic patients: a comparison of severity and outcome. *Diabetes care*, *24*(8), 1433– 1437. https://doi.org/10.2337/diacare.24.8.1433.

[52] Bundó, M., Muñoz, L., Pérez, C., Montero, J. J., Montellà, N., Torán, P., & Pera, G. (2010). Asymptomatic peripheral arterial disease in type 2 diabetes patients: a 10-year follow-up study of the utility of the ankle brachial index as a prognostic marker of cardiovascular disease. *Annals of vascular surgery*, *24*(8), 985–993. https://doi.org/ 10.1016/j.avsg.2010.06.001.

[53] Beckman, J. A., Duncan, M. S., Damrauer, S. M., Wells, Q. S., Barnett, J. V., Wasserman, D. H., Bedimo, R. J., Butt, A. A., Marconi, V. C., Sico, J. J., Tindle, H. A., Bonaca, M. P., Aday, A. W., & Freiberg, M. S. (2019). Microvascular Disease, Peripheral Artery Disease, and Amputation. *Circulation*, *140*(6), 449–458. https://doi.org/10.1161/CIRCULATIONAHA.119.040672.

[54] Morley, R. L., Sharma, A., Horsch, A. D., & Hinchliffe, R. J. (2018). Peripheral artery disease. *BMJ (Clinical research ed.)*, *360*, j5842. https://doi.org/10.1136/bmj.j5842.

[55] Yang, S., Wang, S., Yang, B., Zheng, J., Cai, Y., & Yang, Z. (2017). Alcohol Consumption Is a Risk Factor for Lower Extremity Arterial Disease in Chinese Patients with T2DM. *Journal of diabetes research*, *2017*, 8756978. https://doi.org/10.1155/2017/8756978.

[56] Diabetes UK. Diabetes UK position statement 2020. *Early identification of people with type 2 diabetes*. www.diabetes.org.uk (accessed May 2021).

[57] Burns, P., Gough, S., & Bradbury, A. W. (2003). Management of peripheral arterial disease in primary care. *BMJ (Clinical research ed.), 326*(7389), 584–588. https://doi.org/10.1136/bmj.326.7389.584.

[58] Franz, M. J., Bantle, J. P., Beebe, C. A., Brunzell, J. D., Chiasson, J. L., Garg, A., Holzmeister, L. A., Hoogwerf, B., Mayer-Davis, E., Mooradian, A. D., Purnell, J. Q., Wheeler, M., & American Diabetes Association (2004). Nutrition principles and recommendations in diabetes. *Diabetes care*, 27 Suppl 1, S36–S46. https://doi.org/10. 2337/diacare.27.2007.s36.

[59] Perreault, L., Pan, Q., Mather, K. J., Watson, K. E., Hamman, R. F., Kahn, S. E., & Diabetes Prevention Program Research Group (2012). Effect of regression from prediabetes to normal glucose regulation on long-term reduction in diabetes risk: results from the Diabetes Prevention Program Outcomes Study. *Lancet (London, England), 379*(9833), 2243–2251. https://doi.org/10.1016/S0140-6736(12) 60525-X.

[60] Tuso P. (2014). Prediabetes and lifestyle modification: time to prevent a preventable disease. *The Permanente journal, 18*(3), 88–93. https://doi.org/10.7812/TPP/14-002.

[61] Warren, B., Pankow, J. S., Matsushita, K., Punjabi, N. M., Daya, N. R., Grams, M., Woodward, M., & Selvin, E. (2017). Comparative prognostic performance of definitions of prediabetes: a prospective cohort analysis of the Atherosclerosis Risk in Communities (ARIC) study. *The lancet. Diabetes & endocrinology, 5*(1), 34–42. https://doi.org/10.1016/S2213-8587(16)30321-7.

[62] Emerging Risk Factors Collaboration, Sarwar, N., Gao, P., Seshasai, S. R., Gobin, R., Kaptoge, S., Di Angelantonio, E., Ingelsson, E., Lawlor, D. A., Selvin, E., Stampfer, M., Stehouwer, C. D., Lewington, S., Pennells, L., Thompson, A., Sattar, N., White, I. R., Ray, K. K., & Danesh, J. (2010). Diabetes mellitus, fasting blood glucose concentration, and risk of vascular disease: a collaborative

meta-analysis of 102 prospective studies. *Lancet (London, England)*, *375*(9733), 2215–2222. https://doi.org/10.1016/S0140-6736(10) 60484-9.

[63] Aday, A. W., & Everett, B. M. (2019). Dyslipidemia Profiles in Patients with Peripheral Artery Disease. *Current cardiology reports*, *21*(6), 42. https://doi.org/10.1007/s11886-019-1129-5.

[64] Ridker, P. M., Stampfer, M. J., & Rifai, N. (2001). Novel risk factors for systemic atherosclerosis: a comparison of C-reactive protein, fibrinogen, homocysteine, lipoprotein(a), and standard cholesterol screening as predictors of peripheral arterial disease. *JAMA*, *285*(19), 2481–2485. https://doi.org/10.1001/jama.285.19.2481.

[65] Gurdasani, D., Sjouke, B., Tsimikas, S., Hovingh, G. K., Luben, R. N., Wainwright, N. W., Pomilla, C., Wareham, N. J., Khaw, K. T., Boekholdt, S. M., & Sandhu, M. S. (2012). Lipoprotein(a) and risk of coronary, cerebrovascular, and peripheral artery disease: the EPIC-Norfolk prospective population study. *Arteriosclerosis, thrombosis, and vascular biology*, *32*(12), 3058–3065. https://doi.org/10.1161/ ATVBAHA.112.255521.

[66] Heart Protection Study Collaborative Group (2002). MRC/BHF Heart Protection Study of antioxidant vitamin supplementation in 20,536 high-risk individuals: a randomised placebo-controlled trial. *Lancet (London, England)*, *360*(9326), 23–33. https://doi.org/10. 1016/S0140-6736(02)09328-5.

[67] Pitsavos, C., Panagiotakos, D., Weinem, M., & Stefanadis, C. (2006). Diet, exercise and the metabolic syndrome. *The review of diabetic studies: RDS*, *3*(3), 118–126. https://doi.org/10.1900/RDS. 2006.3.118.

[68] Jellinger, P. S., Handelsman, Y., Rosenblit, P. D., Bloomgarden, Z. T., Fonseca, V. A., Garber, A. J., Grunberger, G., Guerin, C. K., Bell, D., Mechanick, J. I., Pessah-Pollack, R., Wyne, K., Smith, D., Brinton, E. A., Fazio, S., Davidson, M., Zangeneh, F., & Bush, M. A. (2017). American Association of Clinical Endocrinologists and American College of Endocrinology Guidelines for Management of Dyslipidemia and Prevention of Cardiovascular Disease - Executive

Summary. *Endocrine practice: official journal of the American College of Endocrinology and the American Association of Clinical Endocrinologists*, *23*(4), 479–497. https://doi.org/10.4158/EP17 1764.GL.

[69] Ciffone, N. A., & Copple, T. (2019). Managing dyslipidemia for CVD prevention: A review of recent clinical practice guidelines. *The Nurse practitioner*, *44*(1), 8–16. https://doi.org/10.1097/01.NPR. 0000550246.96902.de.

[70] Ong, K. L., Cheung, B. M., Man, Y. B., Lau, C. P., & Lam, K. S. (2007). Prevalence, awareness, treatment, and control of hypertension among United States adults 1999-2004. *Hypertension (Dallas, Tex.: 1979)*, *49*(1), 69–75. https://doi.org/10.1161/01.HYP. 0000252676.46043.18.

[71] Clement, D. L., De Buyzere, M. L., & Duprez, D. A. (2004). Hypertension in peripheral arterial disease. *Current pharmaceutical design*, *10*(29), 3615–3620. https://doi.org/10.2174/13816120433 82819.

[72] Ostchega, Y., Paulose-Ram, R., Dillon, C. F., Gu, Q., & Hughes, J. P. (2007). Prevalence of peripheral arterial disease and risk factors in persons aged 60 and older: data from the National Health and Nutrition Examination Survey 1999-2004. *Journal of the American Geriatrics Society*, *55*(4), 583–589. https://doi.org/10.1111/j.1532-5415.2007.01123.x.

[73] Aboyans, V., Ricco, J. B., Bartelink, M., Björck, M., Brodmann, M., Cohnert, T., Collet, J. P., Czerny, M., De Carlo, M., Debus, S., Espinola-Klein, C., Kahan, T., Kownator, S., Mazzolai, L., Naylor, A. R., Roffi, M., Röther, J., Sprynger, M., Tendera, M., Tepe, G., ... ESC Scientific Document Group (2018). 2017 ESC Guidelines on the Diagnosis and Treatment of Peripheral Arterial Diseases, in collaboration with the European Society for Vascular Surgery (ESVS): Document covering atherosclerotic disease of extracranial carotid and vertebral, mesenteric, renal, upper and lower extremity arteriesEndorsed by: the European Stroke Organization (ESO)The Task Force for the Diagnosis and Treatment of Peripheral Arterial

Diseases of the European Society of Cardiology (ESC) and of the European Society for Vascular Surgery (ESVS). *European heart journal*, *39*(9), 763–816. https://doi.org/10.1093/eurheartj/ehx095.

[74] Lip, G. Y., & Makin, A. J. (2003). Treatment of hypertension in peripheral arterial disease. *The Cochrane database of systematic reviews*, (4), CD003075. https://doi.org/10.1002/14651858.CD00 3075.

[75] Lane, D. A., & Lip, G. Y. (2009). Treatment of hypertension in peripheral arterial disease. *The Cochrane database of systematic reviews*, (4), CD003075. https://doi.org/10.1002/14651858.CD0030 75.pub2.

[76] James, P. A., Oparil, S., Carter, B. L., Cushman, W. C., Dennison-Himmelfarb, C., Handler, J., Lackland, D. T., LeFevre, M. L., MacKenzie, T. D., Ogedegbe, O., Smith, S. C., Jr, Svetkey, L. P., Taler, S. J., Townsend, R. R., Wright, J. T., Jr, Narva, A. S., & Ortiz, E. (2014). 2014 evidence-based guideline for the management of high blood pressure in adults: report from the panel members appointed to the Eighth Joint National Committee (JNC 8). *JAMA*, *311*(5), 507–520. https://doi.org/10.1001/jama.2013.284427.

[77] Sacks, F. M., Svetkey, L. P., Vollmer, W. M., Appel, L. J., Bray, G. A., Harsha, D., Obarzanek, E., Conlin, P. R., Miller, E. R., 3rd, Simons-Morton, D. G., Karanja, N., Lin, P. H., & DASH-Sodium Collaborative Research Group (2001). Effects on blood pressure of reduced dietary sodium and the Dietary Approaches to Stop Hypertension (DASH) diet. DASH-Sodium Collaborative Research Group. *The New England journal of medicine*, *344*(1), 3–10. https://doi.org/10.1056/NEJM200101043440101.

[78] U.S. Department of Agriculture and U.S. Department of Health and Human Services. *Dietary Guidelines for Americans, 2020-2025*. 9th Edition. December 2020. Available at DietaryGuidelines.gov. (Accessed May 2021).

[79] Tóth-Vajna, Z., Tóth-Vajna, G., Gombos, Z., Szilágyi, B., Járai, Z., Berczeli, M., & Sótonyi, P. (2019). Screening of peripheral arterial

disease in primary health care. *Vascular health and risk management, 15*, 355–363. https://doi.org/10.2147/VHRM.S208302.

[80] Lecouturier, J., Scott, J., Rousseau, N., Stansby, G., Sims, A., & Allen, J. (2019). Peripheral arterial disease diagnosis and management in primary care: a qualitative study. *BJGP open, 3*(3), bjgpopen19X101659. https://doi.org/10.3399/bjgpopen19X101659.

[81] Bevan, G. H., & White Solaru, K. T. (2020). Evidence-Based Medical Management of Peripheral Artery Disease. *Arteriosclerosis, thrombosis, and vascular biology, 40*(3), 541–553. https://doi.org/10.1161/ATVBAHA.119.312142.

[82] Steunenberg, S. L., Raats, J. W., Te Slaa, A., de Vries, J., & van der Laan, L. (2016). Quality of Life in Patients Suffering from Critical Limb Ischemia. *Annals of vascular surgery, 36*, 310–319. https://doi.org/10.1016/j.avsg.2016.05.087.

[83] Bhatt, D. L., Steg, P. G., Ohman, E. M., Hirsch, A. T., Ikeda, Y., Mas, J. L., Goto, S., Liau, C. S., Richard, A. J., Röther, J., Wilson, P. W., & REACH Registry Investigators (2006). International prevalence, recognition, and treatment of cardiovascular risk factors in outpatients with atherothrombosis. *JAMA, 295*(2), 180–189. https://doi.org/10.1001/jama.295.2.180.

[84] Khan, S., Flather, M., Mister, R., Delahunty, N., Fowkes, G., Bradbury, A., & Stansby, G. (2007). Characteristics and treatments of patients with peripheral arterial disease referred to UK vascular clinics: results of a prospective registry. *European journal of vascular and endovascular surgery: the official journal of the European Society for Vascular Surgery, 33*(4), 442–450. https://doi.org/10.1016/j.ejvs.2006.11.010.

[85] Osborne, N. H., Upchurch, G. R., Jr, Mathur, A. K., & Dimick, J. B. (2009). Explaining racial disparities in mortality after abdominal aortic aneurysm repair. *Journal of vascular surgery, 50*(4), 709–713. https://doi.org/10.1016/j.jvs.2009.05.020.

In: Peripheral Artery Disease
Editor: Jeremy D. Parks

ISBN: 978-1-53619-968-0
© 2021 Nova Science Publishers, Inc.

Chapter 4

PERIPHERAL ARTERIAL DISEASE: ASSESSMENT TOOLS FOR PRIMARY CARE

Ayla Kara[1,*] and Mehtap Kartal[2]
[1]Ministry of Health Balcova 4th Nusret Fisek Family
Health Center, Izmir
[2]Department of Family Medicine, Faculty of Medicine,
Dokuz Eylul University, İzmir, Turkey

ABSTRACT

The progressive atherosclerotic process is the principal cause of the development of peripheral arterial disease (PAD), and has risk factors in common with atherosclerosis, such as tobacco smoking, diabetes mellitus, dyslipidemia, hypertension and being over the age of 50. The prevalence of PAD, predictably increases with advancing age and the presence of diabetes, leading to a prodigious burden of disease, due to the morbidity and mortality of cardiovascular and cerebrovascular events.

Primary healthcare is an important point of care for the screening of PAD patients, especially those who are asymptomatic. The early recognition of PAD is critically important and the role of the family physician particularly so in the prevention and early assessment of PAD,

---

* Corresponding Author's E-mail: aylkr@hotmail.com.

particularly with regard to risk factors such as diabetes, smoking. To identify at-risk patients in the "murky zone" the physician requires a number of complex approaches in daily work practice. Family physicians can identify these patients using instrumental measurements and if necessary can refer them for further investigation. In the long run, launching an applicable, easy screening program at primary care level makes PAD patients easier to diagnose, leading to earlier diagnosis and treatment, which will significantly improve both the patients' quality of life and life expectancy. In addition to reliable non-invasive diagnostic tests, such as the ankle-brachial pressure index (ABI) simple and easily applied self-assessment tools for the symptoms and performance of patients.

This review focuses on questionnaires for primary care physicians, which can be used for PAD symptom screening, functional impairment and the quality of life of the patients, for example the Edinburgh Claudication Questionnaire (ECQ), Walking Impairment Questionnaire (WIQ), Vascular Quality of Life Questionnaire (VascuQoL), all of which are frequently used by other PAD related disciplines.

Keywords: peripheral artery disease, primary care, Edinburgh claudication questionnaire, walking impairment questionnaire, vascular quality of life questionnaire

INTRODUCTION

In approximately 95% patients, peripheral arterial disease (PAD) is due to atherosclerosis leading to a stenosis (partial) or an occlusion (complete) of the arteries. It occurs in the extremities, usually the lower limbs, due to circulatory disorders of the arteries supplying the limbs. It is a complex and progressive clinical condition with a wide range of clinical presentations, ranging from being totally asymptomatic in its early stages, to developing into necrosis with the threat of amputation of the affected extremity [1].

Diagnostic techniques in patients with PAD should be PAD stage- and patient-oriented, targeted and accurate. Initially, the medical history should be documented and a thorough clinical examination performed with vascular auscultation and palpation [1]. Additionally, there should be a basic examination of the vascular status, including a Doppler ultrasonography of the occlusion pressure in the dorsal pedal and posterior tibial arteries and also, as appropriate, the peroneal artery, in recumbent patients and the calculation of an Ankle-Brachial Index (ABI) [2, 3]. The ABI is the most commonly used noninvasive measurement for the prevalence of asymptomatic PAD among the general population. The cut-off value for the diagnosis of PAD is an ABI value ≤0.9 [2]. This ABI threshold value is derived from epidemiological studies acknowledged in various guidelines issued by the European Society of Cardiology (ESC) [4], the American College of Cardiology/American Heart Association (ACC/AHA) [5], the National Institute for Health and Care Excellence (NICE) [6], and the Transatlantic Inter-Society Consensus (TASC) II [7]. The lower the score the stronger the atherosclerotic changes are in the leg, leading to significant blood-flow obstruction.

There are two clinical classifications of PAD, in terms of symptoms: the Fontaine staging system in Europe and The Rutherford classification in the USA (Table 1). The clinical stages are indicated with the terms "intermittent claudication" (Fontaine stage II) and/or "critical limb ischemia" in later Fontaine stages III and IV [1].

Table 1. Classification of PAD according to Fontaine stages, Rutherford grades and categories [1]

Fontaine Stage	Clinical symptoms	Rutherford		Clinical symptoms
		Grade	Category	
I	Asymptomatic	0	0	Asymptomatic
IIa	Walking distance >200 m	I	1	Mild claudication
IIb	Walking distance <200 m	I	2	Moderate claudication
		I	3	Severe claudication
III	Rest pain	II	4	Rest pain
IV	Ischemic ulcers or gangrene	III	5	Limited ischemic ulceration not exceeding ulcer of the digits of the foot
		III	6	Severe ischemic ulcers or frank gangrene

Pain, typically caused by claudication, implicates reproducible exercise stress-dependent myalgia that improves rapidly within minutes at rest, namely defined as intermittent claudication (IC). Pain affects walking ability, leading to reduced walking performance. This can be described as the measurement of pain-free maximum walking distance and/or impaired walking speed, and when at rest there is still sufficient blood circulation throughout the affected extremities; however, this is not the case for critical limb ischemia (CLI). CLI presents itself with not only pain at rest but also trophic skin and tissue lesions, which points to the loss of balance between arterial perfusion and the metabolic oxygen and nutrient demands of the tissues [1].

Pulse examinations of the lower limbs are helpful, but alone it is insufficient for PAD detection. It is more frequently diagnosed through poor or absent pedal pulses than typical claudication symptoms [7]. Even so, we have to bear in mind that the pulse palpation can be incorrect or inaccurate in over one third of cases, due to various reasons such as clinical error, oedema of the foot or anatomical variations in the vessels. Discomfort due to claudication in the calves can be easily identified, but due to occlusions in the lower-leg or pelvic arteries, exercise stress-dependent pain in the soles of the feet or gluteal region diagnosis can be more difficult solely by clinical examination, especially for the diabetes patients who are identified as being at a higher risk for PAD [1].

In addition to basic examinations of vascular status, there needs to be additional diagnostic tools, namely the Ankle-Brachial Index (ABI). The ABI for each leg equals the ratio of the higher of the two systolic pressures (tibial posterior and anterior artery by doppler ultrasonography) above the ankle, to the average of the right and left brachial artery pressures, unless there is a discrepancy $>=10$ mmHg in blood pressure values between the two arms. In such cases, the higher reading is used for the ABI. The pressure in each leg is measured and the ABIs calculated separately for each leg. In addition to Doppler ultrasound measurements, several other non-invasive techniques have been described for ABI measurements; primarily, these are oscillometric methods [1, 2]. The lower the ABI score, the stronger the atherosclerotic changes in the leg, and blood-flow obstruction is significant. ABI values can be used for PAD severity categorization, as follows: ABI: 0.75–0.9 mild PAD, 0.5–0.75 moderate PAD and severe PAD < 0.5. Nevertheless, the claudication discomfort of the patients may develop with relatively divergent ABI values in different individuals. This is especially so in the case of medial sclerosis, as PAD may be obscured due to normal or increased ABI values [1, 2]. Another detail we should bear in mind is that ABI values of > 0.9 can be found in well-collateralized, proximal high-grade stenoses or occlusions and also with haemodynamically borderline stenoses. In order to detect this, an additional ABI measurement at rest is required immediately after physical exercise, by repetitive tiptoe standing, treadmill (e.g., on a treadmill at 3.2 km/h and 12% incline) or ergometric stress, to increase the PAD sensitivity at rest by 10%. Pain-free and maximum walking distances are documented, as well as walking time and ankle pressure after stress. An ABI decrease of 20% confirms the PAD diagnosis [1, 8]. Throughout this clinical and diagnostic exertions, the focus must be on the patient, as their clinical symptomatology can range from intermittent claudication to critical limb ischaemia and, especially in the presence of comorbid situations, these can result in serious complications such as gangrene and loss of limb organs [6].

All these diagnostic tools focus on determining the severity of the disease, the symptoms of the patients and the functional status, including walking distance and time. Even so, these tools have the disadvantage of being costly and time consuming. They are difficult to carry out in standard clinical situations and are limited at replicating real life performance [9, 10]. It is therefore important to evaluate how the symptoms of PAD patients impact on their daily activities and associated limitations by means of physical functions, such as walking performance, in the physician's daily practice [9]. Therefore, outcomes that present the patients' own perceptions about how PAD affects their daily lives becomes an important issue and one that needs to be assessed. A measurement is needed at this stage, to show patient burden, functional status and quality of life that is easily administered and scored for practical clinical use in the screening and follow up [11, 12]. It would be easier and faster if evaluations were made based on the patients own reports of their real life performance and limitations. Although answers to these self-assessments tools are often provided by the patient, in an attempt to define different aspects of the disease, such as intermittent claudication from the PAD symptoms, this cannot determine its severity or the functional capacity of the patient, as some tools are specific to PAD or acceptable for PAD. In addition to symptoms and functionality, the quality of life of PAD patients also comes to the fore during such procedures.

From among the self-report questionnaires used in PAD studies, we draw specific attention to the WHO/Rose scale, the Edinburgh intermittent claudication Questionnaire (ECQ) scale, the Walking Impairment Questionnaire (WIQ), the Vascular Quality of Life Questionnaire (VascuQoL) scale, and the Intermittent Claudication Questionnaire (ICQ) scale.

When looking at the general properties of the scales, the WHO/Rose and Edinburgh scales define IC, but it does not provide information about its severity. The ECQ includes a response for non-ambulatory patients and a lower-extremity body diagram for patients to indicate leg symptoms indicating IC in multiple locations. The WIQ also focuses on IC while ICQ addresses functional capacity in a more comprehensive framework. The Vascular Quality of Life Questionnaire (VascuQoL) is one of the preferred and recommended health related quality of life questionnaires specific to PAD, while VascuQol-6 (VQ6) also appears to be satisfactory in studies conducted with PAD patients.

If we look at the history of these assessment tools, the Rose Q (WHO) was the first; developed by Geoffrey Rose in 1962. It was a symptom questionnaire to standardize and define claudication, as this was considered to be the only symptom indicating PAD at that time. Developed for epidemiological studies to determine the prevalence of PAD, it was subsequently adopted by the World Health Organization (WHO) in 1968 [13, 14]. In 1992 the Edinburgh Claudication Q (ECQ) was developed, based on the Rose Q/WHO, in order to increase the sensitivity (two questions removed and a diagram added to mark the exact location of pain). This theory reduces the likelihood of an inappropriate response. It was also made shorter and simpler, to increase accuracy. The revised questionnaire includes a body diagram separating claudication into typical and atypical for patients who cannot walk and has been proposed for use in future epidemiological PAD studies [14, 15]. A short while later, in 1996, the San Diego claudication questionnaire (SDCQ) was developed, which includes hip and thigh pain like the ECQ, but evaluates this not only for the right and left leg separately, but for both legs too [16]. While the WHO/ ROSE and ECQ are widely used in Europe, the SDCQ is generally used in studies conducted in the USA. The SDCQ allows for right left leg claudication separation, while the ECQ allows for claudication identification. The SDCQ consists of five possible symptom categories for each leg: Rose claudication, non-Rose exercise calf pain, previously referred to as 'possible IC' and 'probable IC', non-calf exercise leg pain, pain at rest, and no pain [14, 16]. In 1998, McDermott et al. designed the Walking Impairment Questionnaire (WIQ) to measure community-walking ability in patients with PAD and IC [17]. Its scope is therefore appropriately limited to the perspective of health status consists of four subcategories: pain, distance, walking speed, and stair climbing [9, 18]. The WIQ does not cover functional capacity and it is limited to health status related to disability measure due to walking difficulties as correlated with walking distance and speed. Chong et al. developed the Intermittent Claudication Questionnaire (ICQ) in 2002, as a patient-assessed, condition-specific instrument for the assessment of health-related quality of life in intermittent claudication. The ICQ is more comprehensive in the assessment of the functional capacity of a subject with IC, but needs further inclusions regarding self-care and with improved distinction of health status and quality of life items [19]. Comprising 25 items, the VascuQoL was developed in the United Kingdom in 2001, for research purposes [20]. Recently, a short form of the original VascuQol questionnaire has been developed: VascuQol-6 (VQ6) [19]. The VQ6 was developed using a combination of qualitative and quantitative methodology [10, 21].

PAD ASSESSMENT TOOLS THAT FOCUS ON SYMPTOMS

The Rose questionnaire was the first PAD symptom questionnaire to be prepared as a part of the "cardiovascular questionnaire for field use" needed for epidemiological studies [13]. It consists of six questions that define "intermittent claudication," which was thought to be the symptom that indicates PAD. It was subsequently adopted by the World Health Organization (WHO) in 1968 [14]. In 1985, Criqui et al. significantly increased the sensitivity of the WHO/ROSE by expanding the Rose definition of claudication to include possible claudication induced pain, but there was a corresponding decrease in specificity up to 73.1%. At the time, the authors suggested that "hemodynamically significant large-vessel PAD is frequently asymptomatic, although the probability of symptoms increases with the severity of disease. Conversely, symptoms and abnormal pulses do not invariably indicate large-vessel PAD, although the probability increases with the severity of the symptoms" [22].

Developed in 1992, the Edinburgh claudication questionnaire, targets greater sensitivity than the existing WHO/Rose questionnaire to diagnose IC [14]. The Edinburgh Claudication Questionnaire was then developed, based on the WHO/Rose Questionnaire: five questions in the WHO/Rose Questionnaire were either left completely unchanged or only modified slightly; two were omitted, and a diagram was included to allow subjects to mark the exact site of their pain. The new questionnaire is therefore shorter and more straightforward, and its repeatability after an interval of six months was shown to have a kappa value of at least 0.71 in both the clinic and the community patients. Its sensitivity (82.8%) and specificity (100%) was high, and as it was obtained by a physician, the patient history was accepted as a reference [15]. The two studies using revised Rose questionnaires, one is ECQ, have shown a correlation between the reporting of symptoms and non-invasively assessed PAD [15, 22]; however, neither was able to analyze the correlation between subjective reports of leg pain and the presence and extent of ipsilateral PAD. Similar to the ECQ, the San Diego Claudication Questionnaire, which was developed in 1996, included questions on leg-specific (i.e., right versus left) symptoms, thigh and buttock pain, as well as calf pain [15, 22]. In their review, Shorr and Treat-Jakobson remarked that the SDCQ was the most frequently used claudication questionnaire. However, all of the questionnaires were conducted in the United States [22]. The ECQ is used in various countries, translated into different languages such as French, Brazilian Portuguese, Spanish and Turkish and is applied to different ethnicities, such as Black African-Caribbean UK migrants and the Native/Mestizo ethnic group, to include community or primary care settings [22-27].

Claudication questionnaires have undergone several revisions (Table 1) over time depending on the definition of claudication from "typical PAD symptom" to more specific symptom categories beyond classic claudication, and the assessment of leg-specific symptoms. However, sensitivity remains low and specificity is variable. All three questionnaires are seemingly insensitive to PAD detection compared to ABI as a gold standard for diagnosis. Despite all these limitations, current studies are still using ECQ in field surveys or trying to validate it against diagnostic arterial imaging methods such as ABI or Duplex Vascular Ultrasound Scanning [27-29]. The ECQ is an easy-to-use, widely applicable and replicable resource which has good specificity (63.7% and 87.1%, respectively) but too poor a sensitivity (56.2% and 52.5% respectively) to be relied on as a means of diagnosing PAD in primary care [28, 29]. However, a negative ECQ may be used to indicate who does not need to undergo ABI measurement and the application of ECQ under the supervision of a professional can increase its value as a screening tool to evaluate claudication. [30, 31]. Despite these known limitations, the regular use of these assessment tools by family physicians, especially in primary care, can be considered as an opportunity for PAH awareness, diagnosis and monitoring.

Ayla Kara and Mehtap Kartal

Table 2. Evolution of claudication questionnaires [22]

Questionnaire	Year created/ revised	Symptom category	Symptom characteristics
Rose, WHO/Rose	1962	• Intermittent claudication (Rose IC) *Grade 1* *Grade 2*	• Exertional calf pain *Walking uphill or hurrying* *Walking at ordinary pace on the level* • Never starts at rest (standing/sitting) • Never disappears while walking • Causes patient to slow down or stop • Usually disappears in 10 minutes or less
	1985	• Possible IC	Exertional calf pain • Never starts at rest • Otherwise not fully concordant with the Rose IC criteria
	1991	• Probable IC	• Exertional calf pain • One WHO/Rose criteria not fulfilled
ECQ	1992	• Definite IC (Rose IC) *Grade 1* *Grade 2* • Atypical IC	• Fully concordant with Rose IC criteria *Walking uphill or hurrying* *Walking at ordinary pace on the level* • Pain in thigh or buttock in the absence of calf pain, otherwise concordant with Rose IC criteria
SDCQ	1996	• Rose IC • Non-Rose exercise calf pain • Non-calf exercise leg pain • Leg pain on exertion and at rest • No pain	• Fully concordant with Rose IC criteria • Exertional calf pain; at least one Rose IC criteria not fulfilled • Pain in either leg excluding calf (can be thigh or buttock), does not begin at rest • Exertional leg pain starts at rest • Reports no pain in calf, thigh, or buttock

There remains an identifiable need for further questionnaire refinement to increase the sensitivity and correctly identify patients with this disease. This can probably include symptoms differing in location (pain in the hamstrings, feet, shins, joints, or radiating pain in the absence of calf pain) and/or quality (patient reporting symptoms such as tingling, numbness, burning, throbbing, or shooting) compared to those exhibiting classic claudication [13-16, 22]. The ECQ is likely to be accepted as part of a multi-faceted approach to assessing PAD in the community and needs additional diagnostic approaches like ABI in primary care settings in order to allow effective risk factor management [28, 29].

PAD ASSESSMENT TOOLS THAT FOCUS ON FUNCTIONAL IMPAIRMENT

Intermittent claudication is a walking related impairment that specifically worsens after exercise, such as walking or stair-climbing, although it usually disappears after a short rest period [14]. Assessments of the walking ability of PAD patients are important in daily life of patients. Hence, there is a need for a measurement method that can be easily used by patients to determine whether the disease severity has worsened [13-16]. The treadmill exercise test (usually using the Strandness protocol at a speed of 3 km/h and 10% slope) is the conventional test for objective functional assessment and unmasking moderate stenosis, as well as for exercise rehabilitation and follow-up. The test is stopped when the patient is unable to walk due to the initiation of pain or pain intolerance develops, defining distance of walking. A post-exercise ankle SBP decrease >30mmHg or a post-exercise ABI decrease >20% are diagnostic for lower extremity artery disease (LEAD) [1]. However, it does not represent the walking ability of patients during daily life, and this needs treadmill equipment or medical professionals. Moreover, it is not practical in epidemiological research. Validated standardized measures of patient-reported walking capability are needed for not only epidemiological studies but also for interventions studies on functioning in PAD. Therefore, Regensteiner, Hiatt, and others developed the walking impairment questionnaire (WIQ), which makes it simple and easy for patients with PAD and IC to assess walking performance [17, 18, 32]. The WIQ estimates walking distance, walking speed, and stair-climbing capacity in the community. The WIQ evaluates the degree of walking impairment in patients with intermittent claudication on three domains; walking distance, speed, and the ability to climb stairs. For each component, patients rank the degree of difficulty for the corresponding task they were supposed to perform on a Likert scale, which ranges from 4 (no difficulty) to 0 (completely unable to perform the task). Each component of the WIQ was scored according to the procedure described previously [17, 32].

The WIQ can objectively measure PAD symptoms, and its use has been recommended in the Transatlantic Intersociety Consensus [7]. The WIQ has been translated into 38 languages, including Turkish, Dutch, Brazilian Portuguese, Chinese, Korean, Spanish, and is used worldwide [25, 32-37]. Its validation studied with different assessment tools including quality of life measures such as Medical Outcome Study Short-Form 36 (SF-36), RAND-36, EuroQol, European Quality of Life 5 Dimensions (EQ-5D), functional tests Treadmill test, Six-minute walk test (6MWT) and ABI measurement [17, 25, 33-37].

The WIQ also used in intervention studies that evaluate the effect of treatment in patients with peripheral arterial disease [9, 38, 39]. Exercise therapy, namely "supervised exercise programs," in addition to comprehensive secondary prevention, have the potential to benefit patients with PAD by releasing limb symptoms, improving functional capacity, preventing or lessening physical disability, and reducing cardiovascular events [40, 41]. However, it is not always possible for patients to have these programs, as most of the time they are not covered by medical insurance or there is a lack of supervision programs available. Walking exercise at home, after completing a baseline treadmill that will identify coronary ischemia which may develop during a new walking exercise program, three to five times per week, using behavioral change modalities including goal settings and self-monitoring can significantly improves the six-minute walk and treadmill walking performance, physical activity, and patient-reported measures of walking ability [40-42]. Structured home-based exercise (SHE) programs improve the walking ability in PAD patients as showed by improved WIQ score compared to usual care confirming the therapeutic efficiency of the patients' outcomes [38, 39]. As yet, we do not know how effective SHE modalities are for primary care and a simple, well-designed form is also necessary for family physicians to explain and follow up this program, thereby improving both the function and QoL of PAD patients.

The WIQ is a function-specific measure of outcome that does not adequately address the quality of life (QoL) concerns of the patients with claudication. The QoL instruments recommended in all claudication trials and ultimately measurement of QoL, may become the primary endpoint [19].

PAD ASSESSMENT TOOLS THAT FOCUS ON QUALITY OF LIFE (QoL)

Most patients with PAD are asymptomatic; however, other patients may present with a wide array of symptoms that can range from IC to the more severe rest pain and tissue loss associated with CLI. Symptomatic PAD patients can have severe functional limitations that adversely affect their quality of life. This has contributed to the greater awareness and emphasis placed on patient-centered outcomes of functional recovery and QoL in recent years.

Through the developmental process of PAD specific and related assessment tools, generic QoL measures such as Medical Outcome Study Short-Form 36 (SF-36), RAND-36, EuroQol, European Quality of Life 5 Dimensions (EQ-5D) are frequently used for validation studies. Even the Inter-Society Consensus for the Management of Peripheral Arterial Disease (TASC II) [7] recommend use of the physical domains of the generic health-related QoL measure Short Form-36 (SF-36) in addition to the Walking Impairment Questionnaire (WIQ) as patient-based outcome measures for IC in clinical practice.

PAD patients' symptoms range from IC to pain at rest and gangrene, and the natural course of the disease ranges from stable disease with pharmacotherapy to the treatment options needed such as vascular reconstruction or leg amputation. All these different stages of disease and treatment shows the clear need for a reliable and specific quality of life scale that can detect the change in QoL components related to vascular disease, specifically PAD, in clinical studies.

In 2001, the King's College Hospital's Vascular Quality of Life Questionnaire (VascuQol) was designed to be a disease-specific QOL instrument for studies involving patients with lower limb ischemia. For the questionnaire, 25 items were considered with high content validity to be maintained. The questionnaire was easy to complete, taking a mean time of 9.6 minutes. VascuQoL assesses five health domains, namely, pain (four questions), activities (eight questions), symptoms (four questions), emotional (seven questions), and social (two questions). Each question has a seven-point response option, converting the patients' responses to a scale ranging from 1 (worst possible score) to 7 (best possible score) [20]. Responses were averaged for individual domain and composite total scores, giving equal weight to each question and domain. The validation of VascuQoL-25 (VQ-25) has been performed using SF-36 [12]. The disease-specific VascuQol is superior to the generic questionnaires SF–36 and EuroQol-5D with respect to the detection of changes in QoL after follow-up and is recommended for QoL in future trials and the clinical follow-up of PAD patients [43]. Similarly recommended in the Bypass versus Angioplasty in Severe Ischaemia of the Leg (BASIL) trial, the objective of which was to compare the effect on hospital costs and the health-related quality of life (HRQoL) of PAD patients. All VascuQol domains demonstrated sustained improvement over the 36-month time frame, with the largest gains <=3 months after randomization and little change thereafter similar to SF-36 health domains and EQ-5D [44, 45].

In Sweden, the development of the short version, VascuQoL-6 (VQ-6), was based on the psychometric properties of the VQ-25. The VQ6 is a six-item questionnaire, including the most efficient items from the original instrument that demonstrated strong correlations between scores from the original VascuQol and the short version [12, 46, 47]. This short questionnaire is intended to overcome the reluctance to use QoL measures in clinical practice by being easy to administer and quick to complete. It also gives a summary measure, useful as an index, and applicable in vascular registries and has recently been introduced in the Swedish vascular registry [21, 45]. Kumlien et al., tested the VQ6 for content validity, construct validity and test retest reliability, including both quantitative and qualitative methods [12]. Then Larsen et al. evaluated the validity, reliability and responsiveness of the VQ-6 for use in clinical practice and vascular registries and showed that the VQ-6 is a reliable and valid instrument for the evaluation of QoL in patients suffering from PAD in clinical practice, and that the summary score can be used in group comparisons, as in the Swedish vascular registry. It is also emphasized that QoL is an important individual outcome measure not covered by physical measurements of ABI and walking capacity [21]. The VQ6 should be useful in both clinical and research settings due to its multiple benefits, such as good psychometric properties, being easy to use and comprehend by the PAD population, as well as being quick and easy to use, accurate and effective for determining HRQoL. The VQ6 could be a valuable tool for enhancing the understanding of health related QoL in patients with PAD and to guide and to improve treatment strategies in this patient population, especially when translations into different languages are needed. It now looks as if it will soon be in use in several languages, the first one being Brazilian-Portuguese [21] and in different study groups, for interventions showing the minimum important difference and substantial clinical benefit, such as PAD revascularization, different levels of amputations and intermittent negative pressure [49-51].

The patient-assessed intermittent claudication questionnaire (ICQ) evaluated for the properties required of a measure of health outcome by Chong et al., is a condition-specific self-administered instrument for the assessment of health-related quality of life (QoL) in intermittent claudication comparison to the WIQ, the EuroQol, and the SF-36. It is reported to be a practical, reliable, valid, and responsive measure of patient health–related quality of life in the assessment of intermittent claudication on QoL from a patient's perspective, including 16-items, concluding with Cronbach's ∝ of 0.94 scored with the summing up of patient responses to individual items, each of which are equally weighted, and transforming to a 0 to 100 scale, where 0 is the best possible and 100 the worst possible health state [19]. ICQ is also studied together with WIQ for their functional representation according to the World Health Organization's International Classification of Functioning, Disability and Health (ICF) framework. ICF comprehensively describes health-related function and evaluates health status and quality of life measures. The methodology used was ICF-based content assessment to patient-reported vascular disease outcome measures, representing a novel method of assessing such instruments. The study states that the WIQ as can only serve as an assessment of a subject's health status as it pertains to walking disability and it does not address functional capacity or QoL in a significant way. The ICQ, although has a more comprehensive functional assessment of IC, but concept density may obscure meaning [10].

THE ROLE OF PRIMARY HEALTHCARE PROFESSIONALS

Primary healthcare professionals play a key role in the prevention, early diagnosis, referral and follow up of PAD patients. Especially asymptomatic patients with risk factors for PAD having important morbidity and mortality challenges not only for patients but also for physicians. They have to be aware of the needs of PAD patients, including risk factor management, early diagnosis with appropriate tools, and that the coordination of the treatment needs a multi-disciplinary approach.

Throughout the progress of the PAD they need to evaluate their patients, including their symptoms, functional impairment and quality of life. Family physicians can use validated and appropriate instruments, that are easily and quickly applied and implemented and which are acceptable to the patients, and can increase their quality of care by improving symptoms, functioning and the quality of life their patients'. For PAD patients to have a healthier life with fewer complications leading to a better functional status and quality of life, cooperation between family physicians and all PAD related disciplines, such as vascular surgery, endocrinology and cardiology is necessary. The use of patient-reported outcome measures as a common ground with appropriate evidence and guidelines can facilitate the implementing of these tools in their daily practice.

REFERENCES

[1]   Frank, U., Nikol, S., Belch, J., Boc, V., Brodmann, M., Carpentier, P. H., Chraim, A., Canning, C., Dimakakos, E., Gottsäter, A., Heiss, C., Mazzolai, L., Madaric, J., Olinic, D. M., Pécsvárady, Z., Poredoš, P., Quéré, I., Roztocil, K., Stanek, A., Vasic, D. & Terlecki, P. (2019). ESVM Guideline on peripheral arterial disease. VASA. *Zeitschrift fur Gefasskrankheiten*, *48*(Suppl 102), 1–79. https://doi.org/10.1024/0301-1526/a000834. [*Journal of Vascular Diseases*]

[2]   Xu, D., Zou, L., Xing, Y., Hou, L., Wei, Y., Zhang, J., Qiao, Y., Hu, D., Xu, Y., Li, J. & Ma, Y. (2013). Diagnostic value of ankle-brachial index in peripheral arterial disease: a meta-analysis. *The Canadian journal of cardiology*, *29*(4), 492–498. https://doi.org/10.1016/j.cjca.2012.06.014.

[3]   Diehm, C., Lange, S., Darius, H., Pittrow, D., von Stritzky, B., Tepohl, G., Haberl, R. L., Allenberg, J. R., Dasch, B. & Trampisch, H. J. (2006). Association of low ankle brachial index with high mortality in primary care. *European heart journal*, *27*(14), 1743–1749. https://doi.org/10.1093/eurheartj/ehl092.

[4]   European Stroke Organisation, Tendera, M., Aboyans, V., Bartelink, M. L., Baumgartner, I., Clément, D., Collet, J. P., Cremonesi, A., De Carlo, M., Erbel, R., Fowkes, F. G., Heras, M., Kownator, S., Minar, E., Ostergren, J., Poldermans, D., Riambau, V., Roffi, M., Röther, J., Sievert, H. & ESC Committee for Practice Guidelines. (2011). ESC Guidelines on the diagnosis and treatment of peripheral artery

diseases: Document covering atherosclerotic disease of extracranial carotid and vertebral, mesenteric, renal, upper and lower extremity arteries: the Task Force on the Diagnosis and Treatment of Peripheral Artery Diseases of the European Society of Cardiology (ESC). *European heart journal*, *32*(22), 2851–2906. https://doi.org/10.1093/eurheartj/ehr211.

[5] Rooke, T. W., Hirsch, A. T., Misra, S., Sidawy, A. N., Beckman, J. A., Findeiss, L. K., Golzarian, J., Gornik, H. L., Halperin, J. L., Jaff, M. R., Moneta, G. L., Olin, J. W., Stanley, J. C., White, C. J., White, J. V., Zierler, R. E., American College of Cardiology Foundation/ American Heart Association Task Force on Practice Guidelines, Society for Cardiovascular Angiography and Interventions, Society of Interventional Radiology, Society for Vascular Medicine. & Society for Vascular Surgery. (2011). 2011 ACCF/AHA focused update of the guideline for the management of patients with peripheral artery disease (updating the 2005 guideline): a report of the American College of Cardiology Foundation/American Heart Association Task Force on Practice Guidelines: developed in collaboration with the Society for Cardiovascular Angiography and Interventions, Society of Interventional Radiology, Society for Vascular Medicine, and Society for Vascular Surgery. *Journal of vascular surgery*, *54*(5), e32–e58. https://doi.org/10.1016/j.jvs.2011.09.001.

[6] Layden, J., Michaels, J., Bermingham, S., Higgins, B. & Guideline Development Group. (2012). Diagnosis and management of lower limb peripheral arterial disease: summary of NICE guidance. *BMJ (Clinical research ed.)*, *345*, e4947. https://doi.org/10.1136/bmj.e4947.

[7] Norgren, L., Hiatt, W. R., Dormandy, J. A., Nehler, M. R., Harris, K. A., Fowkes, F. G., TASC II Working Group, Bell, K., Caporusso, J., Durand-Zaleski, I., Komori, K., Lammer, J., Liapis, C., Novo, S., Razavi, M., Robbs, J., Schaper, N., Shigematsu, H., Sapoval, M., White, C. & Rosenfield, K. (2007). Inter-Society Consensus for the Management of Peripheral Arterial Disease (TASC II). *European*

journal of vascular and endovascular surgery: the official journal of the European Society for Vascular Surgery, 33, Suppl 1, S1–S75. https://doi.org/10.1016/j.ejvs.2006.09.024.

[8] Rose, S. C. (2000). Noninvasive vascular laboratory for evaluation of peripheral arterial occlusive disease: Part II--clinical applications: chronic, usually atherosclerotic, lower extremity ischemia. *Journal of vascular and interventional radiology: JVIR, 11*(10), 1257–1275. https://doi.org/10.1016/s1051-0443(07)61300-1.

[9] Nicolaï, S. P., Kruidenier, L. M., Rouwet, E. V., Graffius, K., Prins, M. H. & Teijink, J. A. (2009). The walking impairment questionnaire: an effective tool to assess the effect of treatment in patients with intermittent claudication. *Journal of vascular surgery, 50*(1), 89–94. https://doi.org/10.1016/j.jvs.2008.12.073.

[10] C Kauvar, D. S. & Osborne, C. L. (2018). Identifying content gaps in health status measures for intermittent claudication using the International Classification of Functioning, Disability and Health. *Journal of vascular surgery, 67*(3), 868–875. https://doi.org/10. 1016/j.jvs.2017.08.062.

[11] Lindgren, H., Gottsäter, A., Qvarfordt, P. & Bergman, S. (2016). All Cause Chronic Widespread Pain is Common in Patients with Symptomatic Peripheral Arterial Disease and is Associated with Reduced Health Related Quality of Life. *European journal of vascular and endovascular surgery: the official journal of the European Society for Vascular Surgery, 52*(2), 205–210. https://doi.org/10.1016/j.ejvs.2016.05.004.

[12] Kumlien, C., Nordanstig, J., Lundström, M. & Pettersson, M. (2017). Validity and test retest reliability of the vascular quality of life Questionnaire-6: a short form of a disease-specific health-related quality of life instrument for patients with peripheral arterial disease. *Health and quality of life outcomes, 15*(1), 187. https://doi.org/ 10.1186/s12955-017-0762-1.

[13] Rose, G. A. (1962). The diagnosis of ischaemic heart pain and intermittent claudication in field surveys. *Bulletin of the World Health Organization, 27*(6), 645–658.

[14] A Schorr, E. N. & Treat-Jacobson, D. (2013). Methods of symptom evaluation and their impact on peripheral artery disease (PAD) symptom prevalence: a review. *Vascular medicine* (London, England), *18*(2), 95–111. https://doi.org/10.1177/1358863X13480 001.

[15] Leng, G. C. & Fowkes, F. G. (1992). The Edinburgh Claudication Questionnaire: an improved version of the WHO/Rose Questionnaire for use in epidemiological surveys. *Journal of clinical epidemiology*, *45*(10), 1101–1109. https://doi.org/10.1016/0895-4356(92)90150-l.

[16] Criqui, M. H., Denenberg, J. O., Bird, C. E., Fronek, A., Klauber, M. R. & Langer, R. D. (1996). The correlation between symptoms and non-invasive test results in patients referred for peripheral arterial disease testing. *Vascular medicine* (London, England), *1*(1), 65–71. https://doi.org/10.1177/1358863X9600100112.

[17] McDermott, M. M., Liu, K., Guralnik, J. M., Martin, G. J., Criqui, M. H. & Greenland, P. (1998). Measurement of walking endurance and walking velocity with questionnaire: validation of the walking impairment questionnaire in men and women with peripheral arterial disease. *Journal of vascular surgery*, *28*(6), 1072–1081. https://doi.org/10.1016/s0741-5214(98)70034-5.

[18] Myers, S. A., Johanning, J. M., Stergiou, N., Lynch, T. G., Longo, G. M. & Pipinos, I. I. (2008). Claudication distances and the Walking Impairment Questionnaire best describe the ambulatory limitations in patients with symptomatic peripheral arterial disease. *Journal of vascular surgery*, *47*(3), 550–555. https://doi.org/10.1016/ j.jvs.2007.10.052.

[19] F Chong, P. F., Garratt, A. M., Golledge, J., Greenhalgh, R. M. & Davies, A. H. (2002). The intermittent claudication questionnaire: a patient-assessed condition-specific health outcome measure. *Journal of vascular surgery*, *36*(4), 764–864.

[20] Morgan, M. B., Crayford, T., Murrin, B. & Fraser, S. C. (2001). Developing the Vascular Quality of Life Questionnaire: a new disease-specific quality of life measure for use in lower limb

ischemia. *Journal of vascular surgery*, *33*(4), 679–687. https://doi.org/10.1067/mva.2001.112326.

[21] Larsen, A., Reiersen, A. T., Jacobsen, M. B., Kløw, N. E., Nordanstig, J., Morgan, M. & Wesche, J. (2017). Validation of the Vascular quality of life questionnaire - 6 for clinical use in patients with lower limb peripheral arterial disease. *Health and quality of life outcomes*, *15*(1), 184. https://doi.org/10.1186/s12955-017-0760-3.

[22] Criqui, M. H., Fronek, A., Klauber, M. R., Barrett-Connor, E. & Gabriel, S. (1985). The sensitivity, specificity, and predictive value of traditional clinical evaluation of peripheral arterial disease: results from noninvasive testing in a defined population. *Circulation*, *71*(3), 516–522. https://doi.org/10.1161/01.cir.71.3.516.

[23] Lacroix, P., Aboyans, V., Boissier, C., Bressollette, L. & Léger, P. (2002). Validation d'une traduction française du questionnaire d'édimbourg au sein d'une population de consultants en médecine générale [Validation of a French translation of the Edinburgh claudication questionnaire among general practitioners' patients]. *Archives des maladies du coeur et des vaisseaux*, *95*(6), 596–600. [*Archives of heart and blood vessels*]

[24] Makdisse, M., Nascimento Neto, R., Chagas, A. C., Brasil, D., Borges, J. L., Oliveira, A., Gordillo, J., Balsalobre, G., Crozariol, L., Pinho, M., Oliveira, R. & Salles, A. F. (2007). Cross-cultural adaptation and validation of the Brazilian Portuguese version of the Edinburgh Claudication Questionnaire. *Arquivos brasileiros de cardiologia*, *88*(5), 501–506. https://doi.org/10.1590/s0066-782x20 07000500001. [*Brazilian Archives of Cardiology*]

[25] Kara, A., Özçakar, N. & Kartal, M. (2016). Peripheral artery disease reliability and validity study of walking impairment questionnaire. *Nobel Medicus*, *12*(1), 67-73.

[26] Bennett, P. C., Lip, G. Y., Silverman, S., Blann, A. D. & Gill, P. S. (2011). Validation of the Edinburgh Claudication Questionnaire in 1st generation Black African-Caribbean and South Asian UK migrants: a sub-study to the Ethnic-Echocardiographic Heart of

England Screening (E-ECHOES) study. *BMC medical research methodology, 11*, 85. https://doi.org/10.1186/1471-2288-11-85.

[27] Del Brutto, O. H., Sedler, M. J., Mera, R. M., Castillo, P. R., Cusick, E. H., Gruen, J. A., Phelan, K. J., Del Brutto, V. J., Zambrano, M. & Brown, D. L. (2014). Prevalence, correlates, and prognosis of peripheral artery disease in rural ecuador-rationale, protocol, and phase I results of a population-based survey: an atahualpa project-ancillary study. *International journal of vascular medicine, 643589.* https://doi.org/10.1155/2014/643589.

[28] Bendermacher, B. L., Teijink, J. A., Willigendael, E. M., Bartelink, M. L., Büller, H. R., Peters, R. J., Boiten, J., Langenberg, M. & Prins, M. H. (2006). Symptomatic peripheral arterial disease: the value of a validated questionnaire and a clinical decision rule. *The British journal of general practice: the journal of the Royal College of General Practitioners, 56*(533), 932–937.

[29] Boylan, L., Nesbitt, C., Wilson, L., Allen, J., Sims, A., Guri, I., Mawson, P., Oates, C., Stansby, G. & Investigators, O. (2021). *Reliability of the Edinburgh Claudication Questionnaire for Identifying Symptomatic PAD in General Practice. Angiology, 72*(5), 474–479. https://doi.org/10.1177/0003319720984882.

[30] Başgöz, Bilgin Bahadır & TASCI, Ilker & Yildiz, Birol & Acikel, Cengizhan & DEMIRBAS, Seref & Saglam, Kenan. (2016). Sensitivity, Specificity and Predictive Value of the Edinburgh Claudication Questionnaire versus Ankle-Brachial Index for the Diagnosis of Lower Extremity Arterial Disease in Turkish Adults. *Gulhane Medical Journal, 58*, 1. 10.5455/gulhane.173585.

[31] Basgoz, B. B., Tasci, I., Yildiz, B., Acikel, C., Kabul, H. K. & Saglam, K. (2017). Evaluation of self-administered versus interviewer-administered completion of Edinburgh Claudication Questionnaire. *International angiology: a journal of the International Union of Angiology, 36*(1), 75–81. https://doi.org/10.23736/S0392-9590.16.03645-2.

[32] Hiatt, W. R., Hirsch, A. T., Regensteiner, J. G. & Brass, E. P. (1995). Clinical trials for claudication. Assessment of exercise performance,

functional status, and clinical end points. Vascular Clinical Trialists. *Circulation*, *92*(3), 614–621. https://doi.org/10.1161/01.cir.92.3.614.

[33] Verspaget, M., Nicolaï, S. P., Kruidenier, L. M., Welten, R. J., Prins, M. H. & Teijink, J. A. (2009). Validation of the Dutch version of the Walking Impairment Questionnaire. *European journal of vascular and endovascular surgery: the official journal of the European Society for Vascular Surgery*, *37*(1), 56–61. https://doi.org/10.1016/j.ejvs.2008.10.001.

[34] Ritti-Dias, R. M., Gobbo, L. A., Cucato, G. G., Wolosker, N., Jacob Filho, W., Santarém, J. M., Carvalho, C. R., Forjaz, C. L. & Marucci, M. (2009). Translation and validation of the walking impairment questionnaire in Brazilian subjects with intermittent claudication. *Arquivos brasileiros de cardiologia*, *92*(2), 136–149. https://doi.org/10.1590/s0066-782x2009000200011. [*Brazilian Archives of Cardiology*]

[35] Yan, B. P., Lau, J. Y., Yu, C. M., Au, K., Chan, K. W., Yu, D. S., Ma, R. C., Lam, Y. Y. & Hiatt, W. R. (2011). Chinese translation and validation of the Walking Impairment Questionnaire in patients with peripheral artery disease. *Vascular medicine* (London, England), *16*(3), 167–172. https://doi.org/10.1177/1358863X11404934.

[36] Choi, C., Lee, T., Min, S. K., Han, A., Kim, S. Y., Min, S. I., Ha, J. & Jung, I. M. (2017). Validation of the Korean version of the walking impairment questionnaire in patients with peripheral arterial disease. *Annals of surgical treatment and research*, *93*(2), 103–109. https://doi.org/10.4174/astr.2017.93.2.103.

[37] Collins, T. C., Suarez-Almazor, M., Petersen, N. J. & O'Malley, K. J. (2004). A Spanish translation of the Walking Impairment Questionnaire was validated for patients with peripheral arterial disease. *Journal of clinical epidemiology*, *57*(12), 1305–1315. https://doi.org/10.1016/j.jclinepi.2004.03.005.

[38] Li, Y., Li, Z., Chang, G., Wang, M., Wu, R., Wang, S. & Yao, C. (2015). Effect of structured home-based exercise on walking ability in patients with peripheral arterial disease: a meta-analysis. *Annals of*

vascular surgery, *29*(3), 597–606. https://doi.org/10.1016/ j.avsg.2014.10.010.

[39] Parmenter, B. J., Dieberg, G., Phipps, G. & Smart, N. A. (2015). Exercise training for health-related quality of life in peripheral artery disease: a systematic review and meta-analysis. *Vascular medicine* (London, England), *20*(1), 30–40. https://doi.org/10.1177/ 1358863 X14559092.

[40] Hamburg, N. M. & Balady, G. J. (2011). Exercise rehabilitation in peripheral artery disease: functional impact and mechanisms of benefits. *Circulation*, *123*(1), 87–97. https://doi.org/10.1161/ CIRCULATIONAHA.109.881888.

[41] Prévost, A., Lafitte, M., Pucheu, Y., Couffinhal, T. & on behalf the CEPTA educational team. (2015). Education and home based training for intermittent claudication: functional effects and quality of life. *European journal of preventive cardiology*, *22*(3), 373–379. https://doi.org/10.1177/2047487313512217.

[42] McDermott, M. M. (2017). Exercise training for intermittent claudication. *Journal of vascular surgery*, *66*(5), 1612–1620. https://doi.org/10.1016/j.jvs.2017.05.111.

[43] de Vries, M., Ouwendijk, R., Kessels, A. G., de Haan, M. W., Flobbe, K., Hunink, M. G., van Engelshoven, J. M. & Nelemans, P. J. (2005). Comparison of generic and disease-specific questionnaires for the assessment of quality of life in patients with peripheral arterial disease. *Journal of vascular surgery*, *41*(2), 261–268. https://doi.org/10.1016/j.jvs.2004.11.022.

[44] Forbes, J. F., Adam, D. J., Bell, J., Fowkes, F. G., Gillespie, I., Raab, G. M., Ruckley, C. V., Bradbury, A. W. & BASIL trial Participants. (2010). Bypass versus Angioplasty in Severe Ischaemia of the Leg (BASIL) trial: Health-related quality of life outcomes, resource utilization, and cost-effectiveness analysis. *Journal of vascular surgery*, *51*(5 Suppl), 43S–51S. https://doi.org/10.1016/ j.jvs.2010.01.0.

[45] Alabi, O., Roos, M., Landry, G. & Moneta, G. (2017). Quality-of-life assessment as an outcomes measure in critical limb ischemia. *Journal of vascular surgery*, *65*(2), 571–578. https://doi.org/10.1016/j.jvs.2016.08.097.

[46] Nordanstig, J., Karlsson, J., Pettersson, M. & Wann-Hansson, C. (2012). Psychometric properties of the disease-specific health-related quality of life instrument VascuQoL in a Swedish setting. *Health and quality of life outcomes*, *10*, 45. https://doi.org/10.1186/1477-7525-10-45.

[47] Nordanstig, J., Wann-Hansson, C., Karlsson, J., Lundström, M., Pettersson, M. & Morgan, M. B. (2014). Vascular Quality of Life Questionnaire-6 facilitates health-related quality of life assessment in peripheral arterial disease. *Journal of vascular surgery*, *59*(3), 700–707. https://doi.org/10.1016/j.jvs.2013.08.099.

[48] de Almeida Correia, M., Andrade-Lima, A., Mesquita de Oliveira, P. L., Domiciano, R. M., Ribeiro Domingues, W. J., Wolosker, N., Puech-Leão, P., Ritti-Dias, R. M. & Cucato, G. G. (2018). Translation and Validation of the Brazilian-Portuguese Short Version of Vascular Quality of Life Questionnaire in Peripheral Artery Disease Patients with Intermittent Claudication Symptoms. *Annals of vascular surgery*, *51*, 48–54.e1. https://doi.org/10.1016/j.avsg.2018.02.026.

[49] Nordanstig, J., Pettersson, M., Morgan, M., Falkenberg, M. & Kumlien, C. (2017). Assessment of Minimum Important Difference and Substantial Clinical Benefit with the Vascular Quality of Life Questionnaire-6 when Evaluating Revascularisation Procedures in Peripheral Arterial Disease. *European journal of vascular and endovascular surgery: the official journal of the European Society for Vascular Surgery*, *54*(3), 340–347. https://doi.org/10.1016/j.ejvs.2017.06.022.

[50] Ratliff, C. R., Strider, D. & Rovnyak, V. (2019). Quality of Life in Individuals With Peripheral Arterial Disease Who Underwent Toe Amputations: A Descriptive, Cross-sectional Study. *Wound management & prevention*, *65*(4), 34–40.

[51] Mathiesen, I., Seternes, A. & Hisdal, J. (2021). A randomized controlled trial of treatment with intermittent negative pressure for intermittent claudication. *Journal of vascular surgery*, *73*(5), 1750–1758.e1. https://doi.org/10.1016/j.jvs.2020.10.024.

INDEX